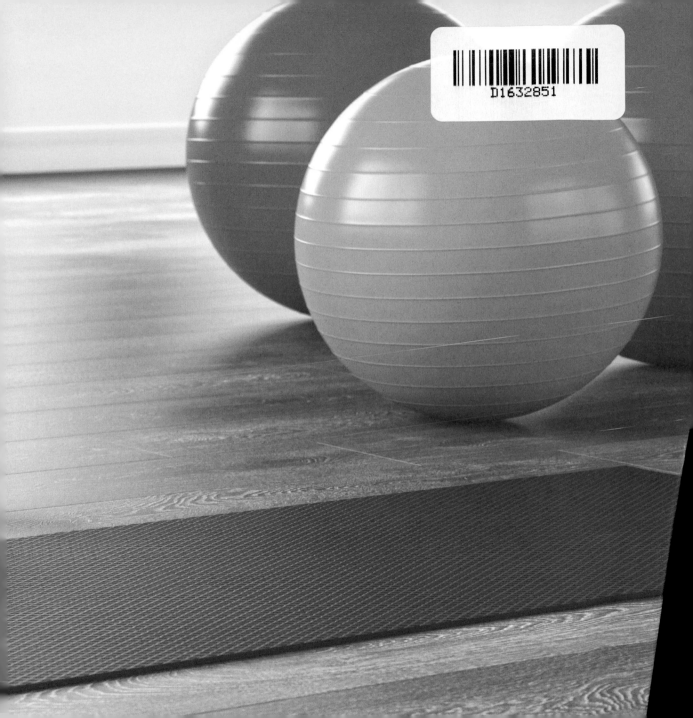

Pilates

A complete guide to total body fitness

igloobooks

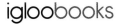

Published in 2015
by Igloo Books Ltd
Cottage Farm
Sywell
NN6 0BJ
www.igloobooks.com

Text and images licensed from Dennis Publishing Ltd
Main image (p.8): iStock

Cover designed by Nicholas Gage
Designed by Stephen Jorgensen
Edited by Natalie Baker

LEO002 1015
2 4 6 8 10 9 7 5 3 1
ISBN 978-1-78557-048-3

Printed and manufactured in China

Contents

How to Use this Book

This guide offers everything you need to practise Pilates at home, from step-by-step instructions to 10-minute workouts. Ready to go? Read these guidelines first to get the most from your practice.

We all lead busy lives which is why *Pilates* has been created to help you shape up quickly, easily and safely. To get the full benefits, it is essential you learn the basics and build up from there. *Pilates* sets out the principles of Pilates with step-by-step photographs and simple instructions.

Take time to read through the book, getting to know the principles and details of the practice. Once you have got the foundations in place and are familiar with the exercises, you can incorporate the workouts into your daily life. Alternatively, dip in and out at your own pace or build your own tailored workouts.

Always do a warm-up before each session, to prepare your body for the workout and help prevent injury. End each session with a cool down and stretch, to relax your body and help it recover for the next session.

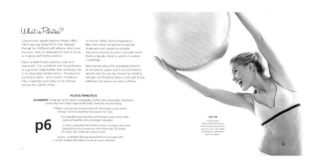

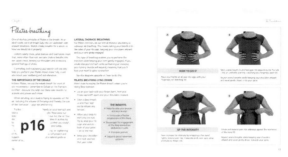

DISCOVER PILATES

Learn about the history of Pilates and why it is hailed as the ultimate exercise system. Discover the benefits it has to offer your body and mind and how it can fit into your busy daily life.

LEARN THE BASICS

Here you will learn the essential breathing and postural techniques that make Pilates effective. You will also learn several key moves that create the foundations of all other Pilates moves.

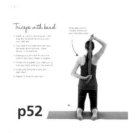

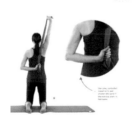

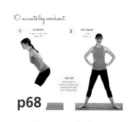

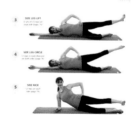

PERFECT THE MOVES

Here you will be guided through each move, step by step, with clear photos and instructions. You will also find modifications for your experience and ability, plus teaching tips to help perfect your alignment.

TRY THE WORKOUTS

You have got the basics, now you can start practising the 10-minute Pilates workouts. Choose them to suit your goals – from sculpting your arms to toning your tummy – or mix and match.

What is Pilates?

German-born Joseph Hubertus Pilates (1883-1967) was way ahead of his time. Plagued through his childhood with asthma, rickets and rheumatic fever, he dedicated the rest of his life to studying and finding wellness.

Pilates studied human anatomy, yoga and martial arts. This, combined with his professions as a gymnast, body builder, diver and boxer, led to his total body transformation – he posed for anatomical charts – and a system of exercise that is hailed by many today as the ultimate exercise for a perfect body.

In the mid 1920s, Pilates emigrated to New York where he opened an exercise studio and soon gained an enviable reputation among the dance and ballet world. Pilates originally called his system of exercise 'Contrology'.

Word spread about the remarkable benefits of his exercise system and it has continued to spread until this very day. Known for building strength and flexibility, Pilates is still used by top ballerinas and dancers as well as athletes.

PILATES PRINCIPLES

ALIGNMENT: If one part of the body is misaligned, it affects the whole body. Working in correct alignment helps improve the body's function and well-being.

BREATHING: Pilates exercises are co-ordinated with the breath to aid control. Breathing is full and relaxed to help power the body.

CONCENTRATION: Focusing the mind and fully committing to each move helps ensure maximum benefits and encourages relaxation.

CONTROL: Every Pilates move is executed with careful control. Knowing what each part of the body is doing allows you to exercise more effectively. The slower the move, the harder you have to work.

FLOW: Using slow, controlled, flowing movements synchronised with the breath enables the body to move as nature intended.

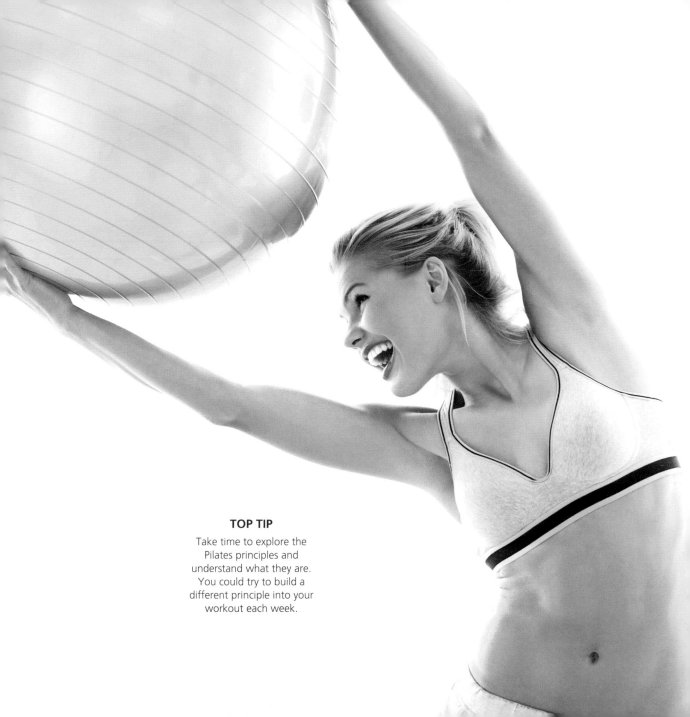

TOP TIP

Take time to explore the Pilates principles and understand what they are. You could try to build a different principle into your workout each week.

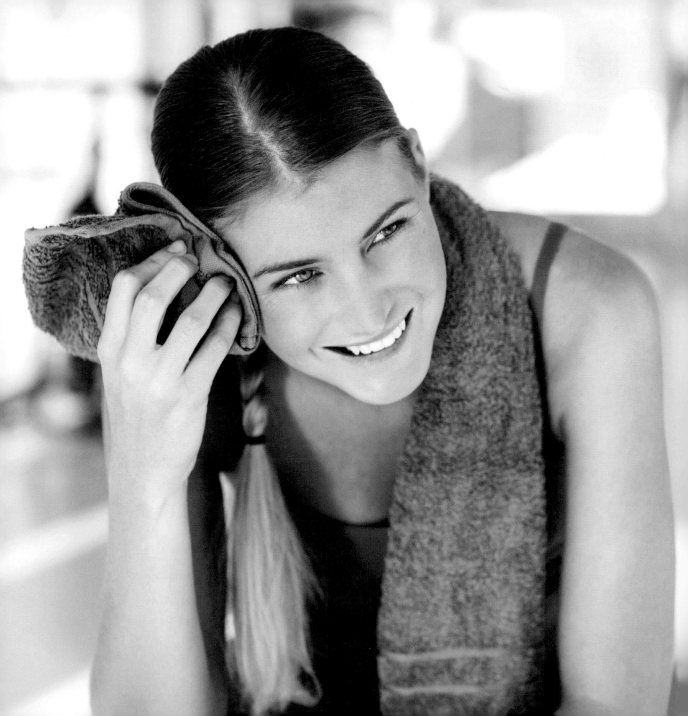

Balance Your Body

Pilates is a body conditioning system of precisely executed exercises that set the body in correct alignment so that muscles can be targeted and exercised effectively. Pilates improves posture, tones and strengthens the body and is known for giving a long, lean look and flat belly.

Pilates is also well known for its benefits as a rehabilitation tool and for helping to protect against injury, aches and pains. It brings the body back into balance through easing tight muscles and strengthening weak ones.

In his pioneering book *Return to Life through Contrology* (1945), Pilates explained that his technique 'develops the body uniformly, corrects wrong postures, restores physical vitality, invigorates the mind and elevates the spirit'.

Studies show that Pilates can strengthen your immune system, protecting you from illness. It can even boost your sex life by strengthening your pelvic floor.

All Pilates exercises begin from your centre or 'powerhouse', helping to develop a strong core. This 'centring' or focusing also helps to connect your mind with your body, shutting out external stress and creating a calming effect.

Today, modern Pilates still teaches the same fundamental exercises but, with time, experts have adapted and modified some of the moves to suit different age groups, body types and goals.

This book uses many of Pilates' original exercises with some variations to help you achieve a strong and toned body, whatever your level of experience.

'In 10 sessions you will feel the difference, in 20 you will see the difference and in 30 you will have a whole new body.'

JOSEPH PILATES

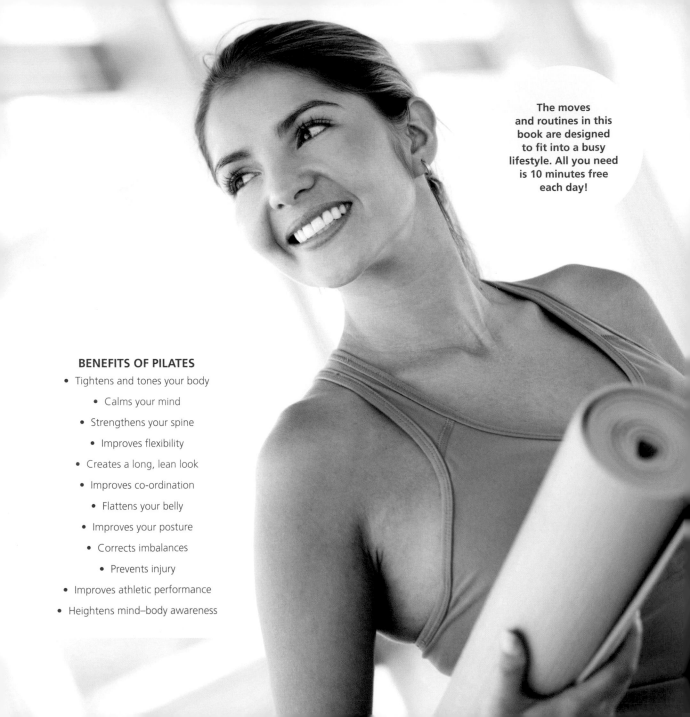

The moves and routines in this book are designed to fit into a busy lifestyle. All you need is 10 minutes free each day!

BENEFITS OF PILATES

- Tightens and tones your body
- Calms your mind
- Strengthens your spine
- Improves flexibility
- Creates a long, lean look
- Improves co-ordination
- Flattens your belly
- Improves your posture
- Corrects imbalances
- Prevents injury
- Improves athletic performance
- Heightens mind–body awareness

Pilates for Modern Life

Modern life is not kind to the human body. Machines have taken over many of the chores that previous generations cursed, such as scrubbing floors and clothes, or walking or cycling to work in the rain and snow. While it is wonderful that we don't have to endure these hardships, the cost to our bodies has been huge and our posture, weight, health and well-being have suffered enormously as a result.

Sitting at computers, desks and cars has given us hunched backs, round shoulders and fat stomachs. Slumping on the sofa watching TV has given us weak backs, flabby bottoms and poor circulation. These factors lead to back and neck pain, headaches and increased stress caused by poor breathing.

GOOD FOR POSTURE

Pilates can help to address many modern ailments and is routinely prescribed by physiotherapists, doctors and osteopaths as a remedy for back, shoulder, postural and joint problems. The precise, controlled nature of Pilates makes the exercises extremely safe for everyone and the focus on body and joint alignment can help undo postural problems.

Many issues that people take to their GP, including back and neck pain and urinary incontinence, can be rectified with regular Pilates exercises. It strengthens where the body is weak and lengthens where it is tight. Developing core strength helps prevent back pain and enables the body to move more freely. Pilates also ensures the spine is regularly moved safely through all of its natural range of motion – flexion, extension and rotation help it stay supple and strong.

Pilates is written with our busy modern lives in mind – in spite of our time-saving machines, we've probably never been more time deprived! The moves and routines in this book are designed to fit into your lifestyle, no matter how full your day.

TAKE 10 MINUTES

Almost everyone can find 10 minutes in a day and those precious moments will help you to stay strong and supple. The moves in this book can be performed anywhere – in your office at lunchtime or beside your bed at night. What matters is that you actually DO the exercises to help you get the most out of your busy life and keep your body and mind young and flexible!

CHAPTER 1

The Foundations

The following pages are the most important in this book. You will learn the fundamental foundations of Pilates on which you will build your practice.

Over the course of these pages, you will learn the correct posture, breathing and alignment you need to practise Pilates.

You will also learn about your core and why it is key to good health. It is said that the best things in life come to those who wait and this is true with Pilates!

The Pilates breath can take more than a few sessions before it starts to feel natural as most of us have forgotten how to breathe properly.

You might find you are holding your breath when you are doing the exercises. If so, just relax, follow the instructions and remember that practice makes perfect!

Pilates posture

As you read this page, take a minute to check your posture. Are you sitting up straight or slumped on the sofa or over a desk? For most of us, good posture is tiring to maintain for more than a few minutes. Our modern day lifestyle has weakened our postural muscles and put our bodies out of alignment. Poor posture not only leads to fatigue and backache, it makes you appear shorter and rounder, too.

Try standing tall with your shoulders open, your abdominals pulled slightly in and breathe more deeply. You will instantly notice that you look taller with a flatter stomach. You will also feel more alert and energised. Ideally, this is how we should all carry ourselves – and this is what Pilates can help you achieve.

Practise Pilates regularly and you will notice that you start to sit naturally and stand taller without any effort. Pilates can give you the natural poise and elegance of a dancer. But first you need to learn the basics.

HOW TO FIND PERFECT POISE

Stand sideways on to a mirror and be honest with yourself! Try to adopt your usual posture, then compare it with the photo on the opposite page (far right). Don't try to adopt a very different posture immediately as this will feel unnatural and may strain certain muscles. Just identify your weaknesses, such as round shoulders or pot belly, and feel grateful that you are about to improve them!

A quick fix for all posture types is to imagine that you have a string coming from the top of your head and that an invisible force is pulling that string up. Try this now. Stand in your usual posture, sideways to a mirror. Now draw your whole body upwards imagining that string, then check the mirror again. It is simple but effective!

TOP TIP

Improve your posture by drawing up, stretching the tips of your ears from your feet while relaxing your shoulders back and down.

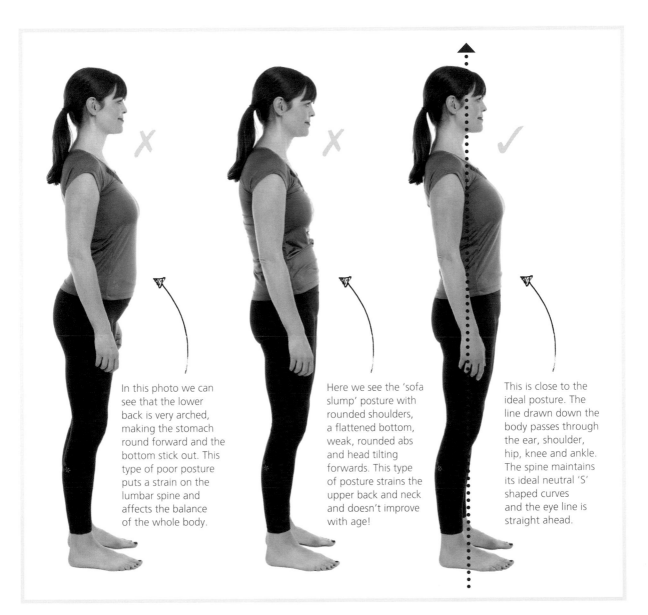

In this photo we can see that the lower back is very arched, making the stomach round forward and the bottom stick out. This type of poor posture puts a strain on the lumbar spine and affects the balance of the whole body.

Here we see the 'sofa slump' posture with rounded shoulders, a flattened bottom, weak, rounded abs and head tilting forwards. This type of posture strains the upper back and neck and doesn't improve with age!

This is close to the ideal posture. The line drawn down the body passes through the ear, shoulder, hip, knee and ankle. The spine maintains its ideal neutral 'S' shaped curves and the eye line is straight ahead.

Pilates breathing

One of the key principles of Pilates is the breath. In an ideal world, we would all breathe fully into our abdomen with relaxed shoulders.

Unfortunately, stress, poor posture and bad habits mean that, more often than not, we take shallow breaths into our upper chest, tensing our shoulders and increasing general feelings of stress. Controlling and maximising your breath will not only help you perform your Pilates moves more fully, it will also boost your well-being and aid relaxation.

THE IMPORTANCE OF THE EXHALE

In basic Pilates, we use the exhale breath for most movements because this helps our deep core muscles to activate and power each move.

Try this: Stand up, place your hands on your stomach and take a deep breath in, relaxing your abs. Now blow out and keep blowing out ALL the air. You should feel your deep abs tighten and draw in as they try to expel the air. Your abs contract to force the air out of your lungs.

This natural 'flattening' or 'tightening' of the abs as we exercise will protect and support our spine and help to build a natural girdle or corset of strength.

PILATES BREATHING LYING DOWN

Here's how to employ the Pilates breath when you are doing floor exercises.

Try this: Lie on your back with your knees bent, feet and knees hip-width apart and your shoulders relaxed. Take a deep breath in and then 'sigh' out to release any tension.

Allow your body to melt into the mat. Try to relax your rib cage and sacrum on to the mat. Relax your shoulders and neck and feel that your collar bones are wide and flat.

Inhale and imagine your rib cage expanding without allowing your back to arch or your ribs to lift off the mat. Breathe in through your nose and out through your mouth to help you to engage your core.

Take several breaths in and when you are comfortable, try the breathing while keeping a gentle contraction of navel to spine.

THE BENEFITS
- Helps to relax your muscles and ease tension
- Encourages effective oxygenation of the blood
- Encourages the engagement of the deep transversus abdominis muscle
- Improves posture
- Supports good movement patterns
- Focuses the mind

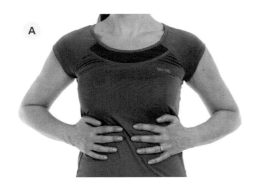

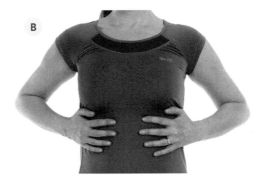

HOW TO DO IT

Place your hands on to your rib cage with your fingertips just touching (A).

Take a deep breath in and feel your ribs expand out to the side, pushing your fingertips apart (B).

Repeat several breaths while keeping your shoulders relaxed and navel gently drawn in to your spine.

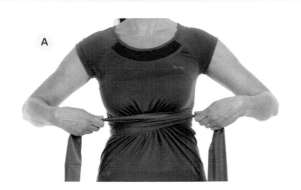

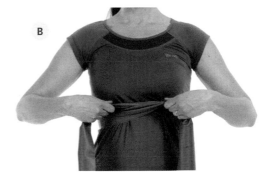

UP THE INTENSITY

Now increase the intensity by wrapping a resistance band tightly around your ribs. Cross the ends over each other and hold as shown (A).

Inhale and expand your ribs sideways against the resistance of the band (B).

Repeat several breaths while keeping your shoulders relaxed and navel gently drawn towards your spine.

Finding neutral

In Pilates we talk about a neutral spine. But what does neutral really mean? Your spine is made up of 24 articulating vertebrae which should form a nice gentle 'S' shape rather than the '?' shape of a hunched upper back and flat lower back that we see so often these days.

This 'S' shape is your spine's neutral position and when in correct alignment, it provides natural shock absorption from impact, allowing the weight of your body to be transferred through the centre of each joint. However, if your body is out of alignment, its weight will be displaced, and put a strain on your vertebrae and joints.

A neutral spine and pelvis enables your limbs to move freely and naturally. If, for example your pelvis is tilted forwards this can affect the muscles of your back, bottom and thighs and can lead to weakness, tightness and injury.

Many Pilates exercises are performed in neutral. However, some moves require you to imprint your spine on the floor instead to create a safer position for challenging your abs.

FIND A NEUTRAL SPINE LYING DOWN

1. Lie with your knees bent and feet hip-width apart. Press your lower back flat on the floor.

2. Arch your lower back off the floor. Continue four or five times, making the movements smaller and smaller.

3. Finally, settle at a point where your back is neither flat on the floor or arched off the floor but in-between.

TOP TIP
Imagine you have a big bowl of soup on your stomach. You don't want the soup to tip out of the front or back of the bowl but to lie flat.

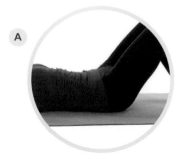
A

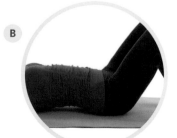
B

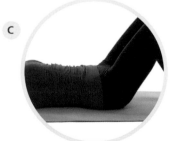
C

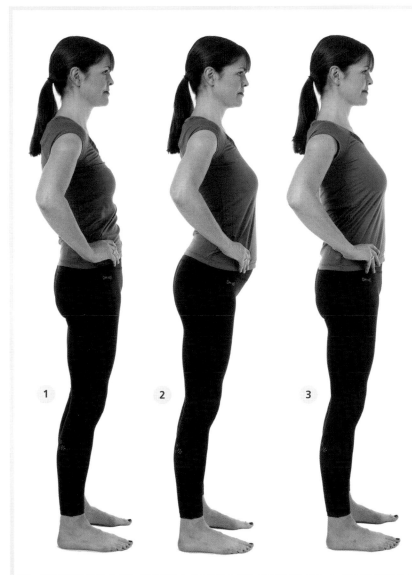

FIND NEUTRAL IN STANDING

Stand with your feet hip-width apart and knees soft.

1. First tuck your tail bone under, flattening out your lower back.

2. Now arch your back by sticking your bottom out. Move four to five times in each direction making the movements smaller and smaller until you come to rest in the middle.

3. Your back should have a gentle curve. If you place your hands on your pelvis you will feel that your pubic bone is in line with your hip bones. Check your stomach – if you arch your back too much, your stomach will poke out.

Your shoulders should also be in a neutral position, with the shoulder blades drawn slightly towards each other and down.

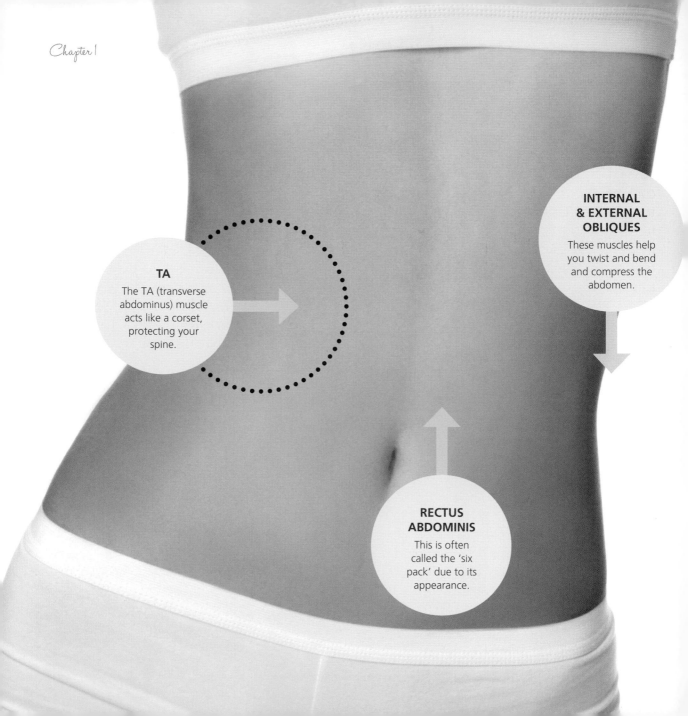

INTERNAL & EXTERNAL OBLIQUES

These muscles help you twist and bend and compress the abdomen.

TA

The TA (transverse abdominus) muscle acts like a corset, protecting your spine.

RECTUS ABDOMINIS

This is often called the 'six pack' due to its appearance.

About your core

Your core is the centre of your body and comprises all the muscles in and around your trunk. Having a strong core is key to a healthy, functional body. The stronger your core is, the more weight you can lift with your arms, the more power you can push through your legs and the more stable your spine and pelvis are.

All Pilates movements begin at the core. By connecting to your deep core muscles when exercising, your pelvis and spine will be supported, helping to prevent injury. Strengthening your core with Pilates tones all the layers of muscles around your mid section, drawing in your waist, flattening your tummy and strengthening your pelvic floor.

HOW TO CONNECT

We're all familiar with the rectus abdominis muscle, commonly known as the six pack muscle. This is the most superficial ab muscle and consists of two vertical bands of muscle which flex your spine, bringing your chest towards your hips and vice versa. Beneath this lies the internal and external oblique muscles, which run diagonally and allow your spine to side bend and twist.

Deeper still lies the transversus abdominis (TA) which is like a corset that wraps around your waist. This muscle draws your navel in towards your spine. The TA does not move your spine but supports it. The TA works in harmony with another set of deep core muscles, collectively known as the pelvic floor. These muscles are shaped like a sling and offer support for your pelvis and internal organs. You might have already discovered these muscles if you have ever tried to stop yourself from going to the loo or if you have had a baby and have practised post-natal pelvic floor exercises.

ZIP IT UP

In this book, you will be reminded to 'draw navel to spine' – this action should feel as if you are gently drawing your pelvic floor upwards and your tummy button inwards as if you are zipping up a tight pair of jeans. This action will flatten your tummy and stabilise your spine and pelvis. Each Pilates exercise should begin from your core and you will be instructed to 'inhale to prepare... exhale and engage navel to spine' as you flow into your exercise. It may feel unnatural to begin with, but practice makes perfect!

Basic moves

The following Pilates exercises lay the foundations for many of the moves in this book. It is important to be familiar with them first. They will take your spine through flexion, extension and rotation and mobilise your shoulders, opening your chest and strengthening your core.

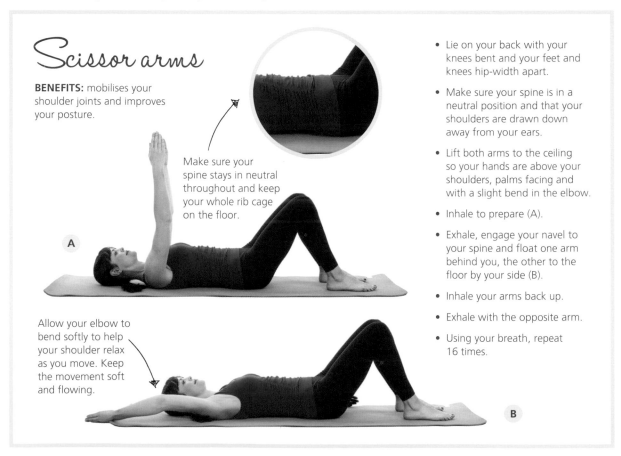

Scissor arms

BENEFITS: mobilises your shoulder joints and improves your posture.

Make sure your spine stays in neutral throughout and keep your whole rib cage on the floor.

A

Allow your elbow to bend softly to help your shoulder relax as you move. Keep the movement soft and flowing.

- Lie on your back with your knees bent and your feet and knees hip-width apart.

- Make sure your spine is in a neutral position and that your shoulders are drawn down away from your ears.

- Lift both arms to the ceiling so your hands are above your shoulders, palms facing and with a slight bend in the elbow.

- Inhale to prepare (A).

- Exhale, engage your navel to your spine and float one arm behind you, the other to the floor by your side (B).

- Inhale your arms back up.

- Exhale with the opposite arm.

- Using your breath, repeat 16 times.

B

Spinal twist

BENEFITS: mobilises your spine, particularly your thoracic spine (upper back), improves your posture and stretches your shoulders and chest.

- Lie on your right side, with your knees bent, fingertips touching in front, hips stacked on top of one other. Keep your waist hollow (A).

- Inhale and reach your top arm to the ceiling (B).

- Exhale and reach back towards the floor behind you, keep your waist and hips still and let your head and eyes follow the move (C).

- Inhale into your ribs and hold the open position.

- Exhale, draw your navel to your spine and bring your arm back to the start.

- Repeat four times on each side. On the final rep, hold the open position for three deep breaths.

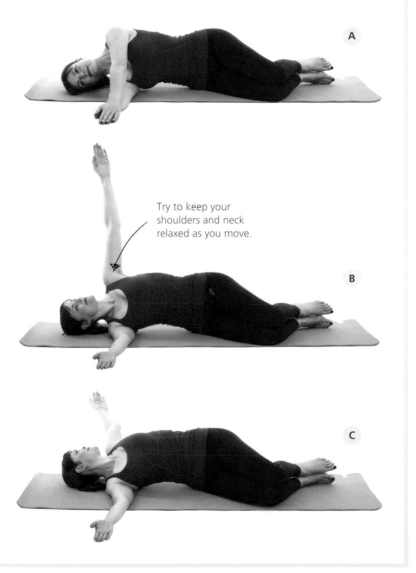

A

Try to keep your shoulders and neck relaxed as you move.

B

C

Pelvic tilt

BENEFITS: mobilises your lumbar spine, flattens your abs and strengthens your pelvic floor and core.

- Lie on your back with your knees bent with your feet and knees hip-width apart and spine in neutral. Inhale to prepare (A).

- Exhale and draw your pelvic floor up and your navel in as you tuck your tail bone under. At the same time press your lower back into the floor (B).

- Inhale and lengthen back into a neutral position.

- Continue for 10 to 15 breaths.

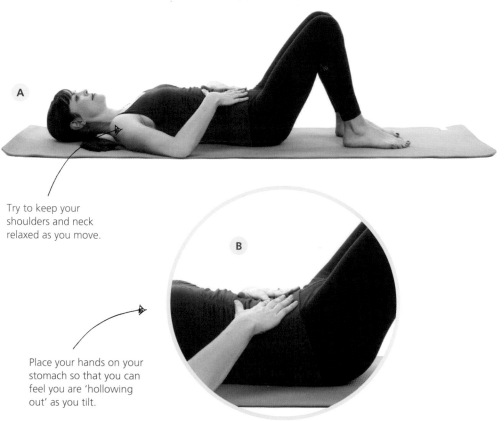

Try to keep your shoulders and neck relaxed as you move.

Place your hands on your stomach so that you can feel you are 'hollowing out' as you tilt.

Basic ab curl

BENEFITS: strengthens your core and flattens your abs.

Try to keep your pelvis very still and your thighs and pelvis relaxed or your legs might try to 'help you' by taking the emphasis off your abs.

- Lie on your back with your knees bent and feet and knees hip-width apart.
- Begin in neutral spine with your shoulders drawn away from your ears.
- Inhale and gently lengthen the back of your neck, tucking your chin slightly (A).
- Exhale, engage your navel to your spine and draw your shoulder blades down as you contract your abs. Fold your head and shoulders off the mat while reaching your fingers down to your toes. Keep your arms off the mat (B).

- Inhale and maintain your navel to spine connection as you take a shallow breath into the sides of your ribs.
- Exhale and return your head, shoulders and arms to the mat.
- Using your breath, do eight reps.
- To progress, on the final repetition, stay in the 'up' position and add 12 crunches, exhaling each time you lift a little higher off the floor.

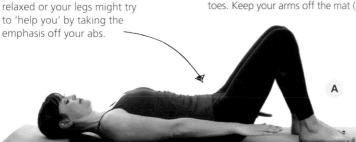

A

If you feel your neck is straining, place one hand behind your head to gently support its weight.

Bring your rib cage towards your hip bones as you lift.

B

VARIATIONS

1. Place a pillow or ball between your knees and squeeze as you curl up.

2. Place both hands behind your head.

3. Place both hands in front of your head with your fingertips touching your temples.

4. In the 'up' position, lift both arms up so your upper arms are beside your ears, maintaining the ab crunch. This is an advanced move.

Table-top legs

BENEFITS: stabilises your pelvis and spine and strengthens your core.

- Lie on your back with your knees bent and feet and knees hip-width apart with your spine and pelvis in neutral.

- Exhale and engage your navel to your spine, keeping your hips still as you lift one leg so your knee is above your hip and bent to 90° like the leg and top of a table (A).

- Inhale and keep a stable spine and pelvis as you lower your foot to the lift-off spot.

- Repeat on the other side and continue alternating your legs for 12 reps.

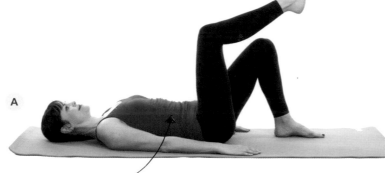

A

This exercise might seem very simple, but the challenge is to keep a neutral spine and flat tummy throughout, while preventing your hips from rolling from side to side.

TO PROGRESS

To progress, do as above, but lift one leg and then the other one on exhale. Inhale to hold in a table top then exhale to lower one leg then the other on a second exhale. Keep your spine very still as you lift and lower your second leg.

Basic breast stroke

BENEFITS: mobilises your spine, particularly your thoracic spine or upper back and strengthens your postural muscles around your shoulder girdle.

Use the muscles of your spine to lift you and use your arms to assist only.

Keep the full weight of your legs on the mat.

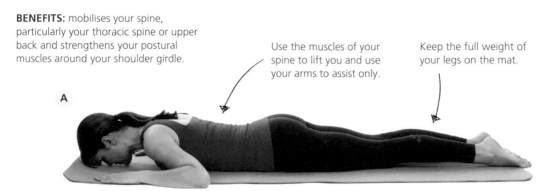

A

- Lie on your stomach with your legs drawn together and your arms bent on the floor – fingertips approximately in line with your nose (A).

- Inhale to prepare.

- Exhale and gently draw your navel to your spine as you push your hands into the floor and draw your shoulder blades down, away from your ears.

- At the same time extend your head and shoulders off the floor while keeping your bottom rib in contact with the floor (B).

- Inhale to hold up and try to lengthen the front of your chest away from your toes.

- Exhale to lower yourself back to the start.

- Repeat eight times.

Try to lengthen your spine as you lift and lower. Always keep your head and neck following the line of your spine.

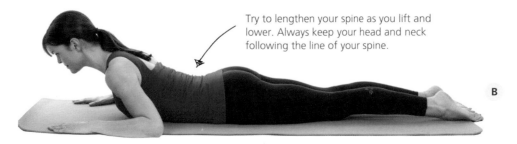

B

The workouts

Now you have learned the basics, you are ready for a daily workout. In this section you will find the moves to tone up all over and improve your well-being. This book is divided into sections to target your trouble zones: bum, arms, legs, abs and back.

For those days when you are 'in the zone', do a few workouts together. Begin with the warm up then try the Arms, followed by the Legs and Abs moves for a 30-minute session. These gentle exercises can be performed every day. The most important thing is to listen to your body! Remember the principles of Pilates and if you can't complete an exercise with great form or you are losing concentration and flow – stop!

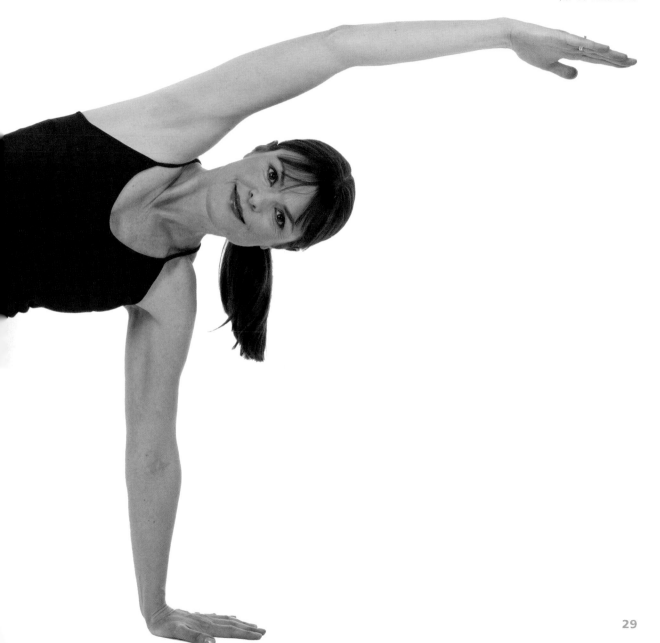

Pilates kit

All you need to practise Pilates is your body and your mind! However, a few pieces of clothing and equipment can help support your body and ensure you get the maximum results from your workouts.

Ideally, you will have a Pilates or yoga mat but, if not, you can fold a blanket so you have some form of cushioning underneath you during the floor exercises. Make sure you have enough space to move freely and wear comfortable, breathable clothing.

You can also use a resistance band. This simple but effective tool adds resistance to your exercises to increase the challenge and build your strength. Resistance bands come in three different strengths. A medium resistance band works well for these exercises. However, if you are recovering from a shoulder injury, begin with a gentle resistance band.

A couple of the exercises use dumbbells. If you don't have any, you can use small bottles of water or cans of beans instead.

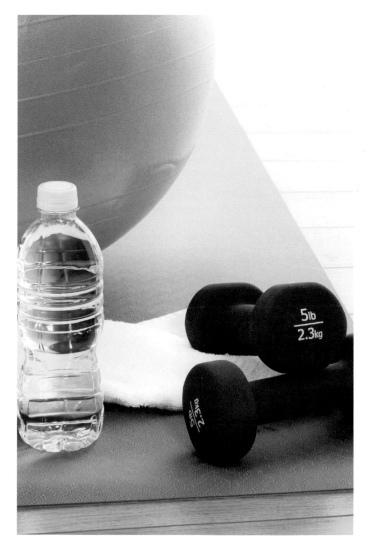

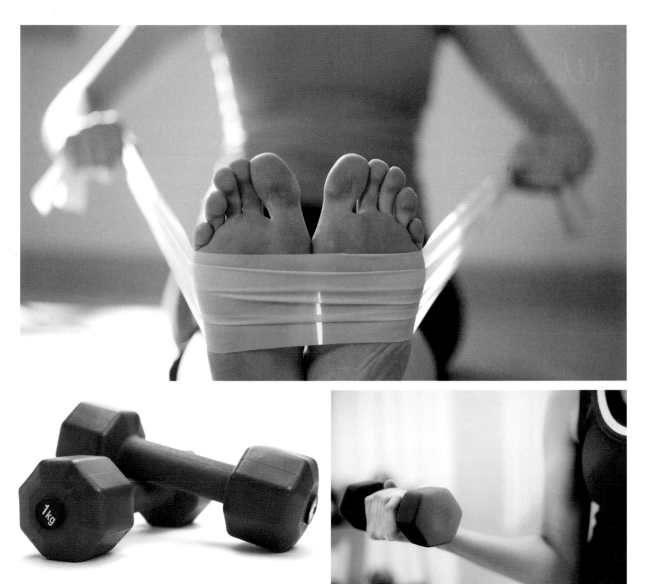

Warm up

Before you begin your Pilates exercises you need to prepare your body, so a good warm up is essential. These exercises are designed to prime and prepare your whole body for exercise, increasing blood flow to your muscles and warming up your joints. The warm up only takes a couple of minutes. If it is cold, or you are just out of bed or are feeling a little stiff, it is a great idea to repeat the circuit twice.

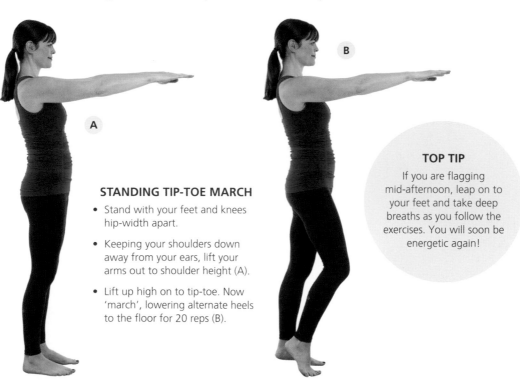

STANDING TIP-TOE MARCH

- Stand with your feet and knees hip-width apart.

- Keeping your shoulders down away from your ears, lift your arms out to shoulder height (A).

- Lift up high on to tip-toe. Now 'march', lowering alternate heels to the floor for 20 reps (B).

TOP TIP

If you are flagging mid-afternoon, leap on to your feet and take deep breaths as you follow the exercises. You will soon be energetic again!

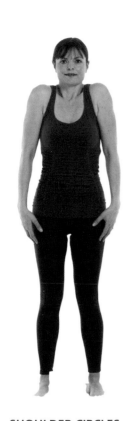

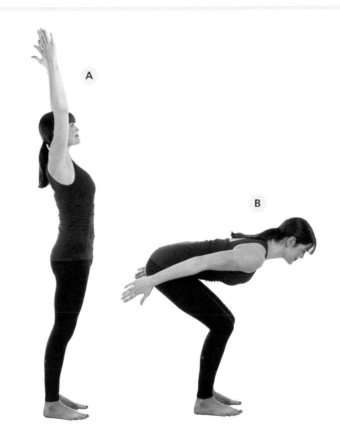

SHOULDER CIRCLES

- Stand with a tall posture and neutral spine.

- Circle your shoulders backwards 10 times, finishing with them open and your shoulder blades drawn gently back and down.

SKIING

- Stay standing as in the exercise opposite. Inhale to reach your arms up high overhead (A).

- Exhale to bend your hips and knees into a skiing position, swinging your arms back behind you (B).

- Inhale and reach arms back up overhead.

- Continue in time with your breath for 20 reps.

CHAPTER 2

Tone Your Bum

Your bottom contains one of the largest muscles in your body – the gluteus maximus. Known as a 'global' muscle, it is responsible for creating movement. Beneath it are lesser known muscles, called 'local' or 'stabiliser' muscles that help stabilise your pelvis. Pilates works both global and local muscles, helping your body to move as nature intended and keeping it strong and balanced with a firm bottom as a bonus!

Sitting on your behind for a large part of the day can create a weak and flabby bum. Pilates can help prevent this. For a strong and functioning behind, focus on each movement and think about the muscle that's working.

These exercises work on strengthening your glutes and hamstrings as well as the stabiliser muscles of your bottom and hips. Pay attention to the training tips since a very simple adjustment, such as rotating your foot and leg outwards, will make a big difference to the results.

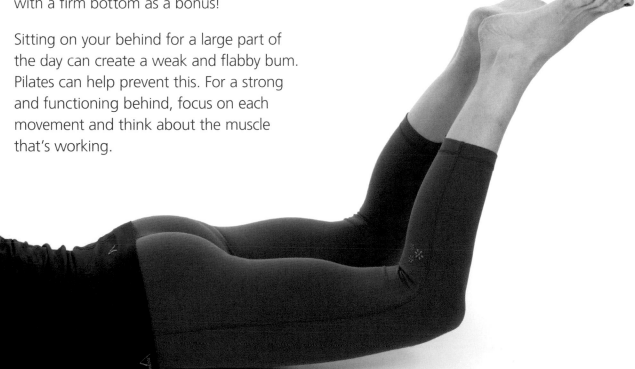

Crab walk

- Stand with your feet and knees hip-width apart. Tie a band around your legs just above your ankles ensuring there is no slack in this position (A). Place your hands on your hips and draw your shoulders back and down.

- Take 10 steps to the right, keeping your upper body still – no rocking (B)!

- Take 10 steps back to the left. Now rotate your legs outwards so that your toes point out to the sides and repeat 10 steps each way (C).

- Finally rotate your legs inwards so that your toes turn in and repeat 10 steps each way (D).

- As you get stronger and if time allows, you can perform two to three sets of each of the exercises.

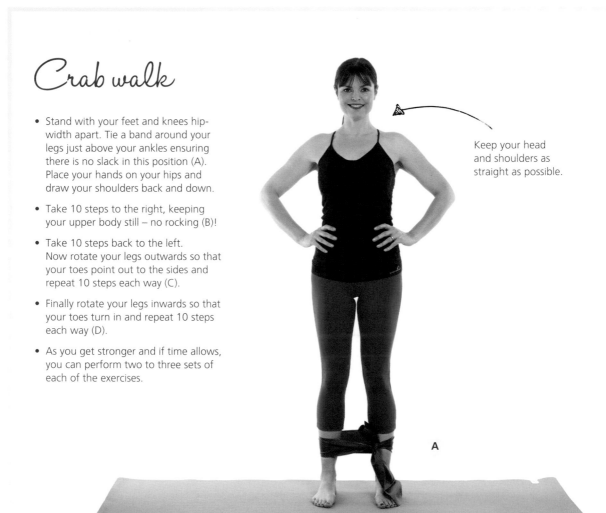

Keep your head and shoulders as straight as possible.

A

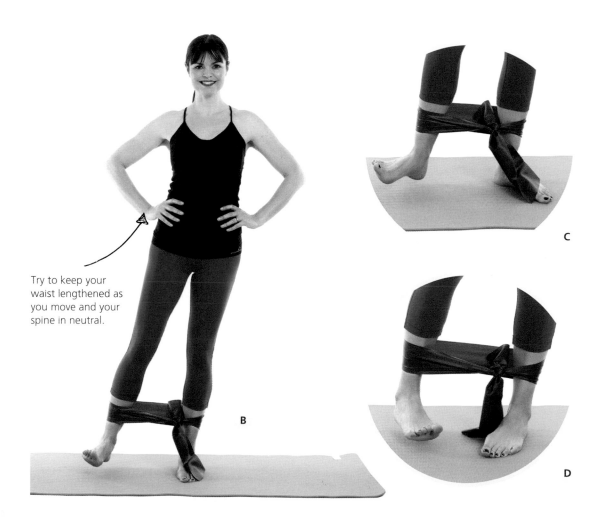

Try to keep your
waist lengthened as
you move and your
spine in neutral.

B

C

D

Oyster 1 & 2

PART 1

- Lie on your right side, with your head on your outstretched arm and both knees bent (A).

- Exhale, engage navel to spine and open your left knee – like a book opening – keeping your hips still and stacked (B).

- Inhale to close.

- Repeat 12 times.

Keep your hips stacked one on top of the other.

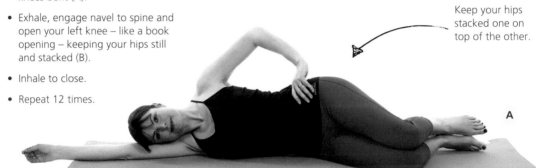

A

Keep your core engaged so that the weight of your waist is slightly drawn off the floor.

Make sure that your top hip stays completely still as you open.

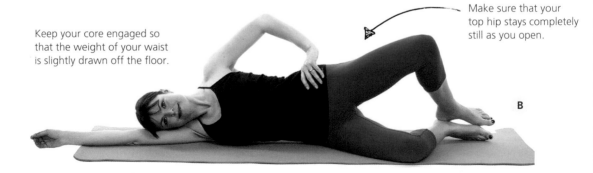

B

PART 2

- Now repeat the same exercise but this time lift both feet off the floor with each repetition (C).

- Complete 12 repetitions.

- Now change to your left side and repeat part 1 and 2 on your right leg.

TO PROGRESS

- Tie the resistance band around your knees with just a little slack in the closed position.

- Repeat the steps above against the resistance of the band.

C

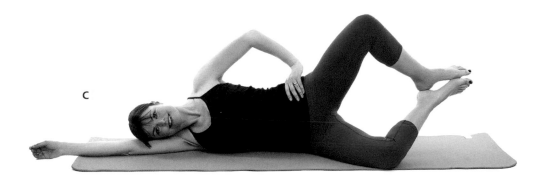

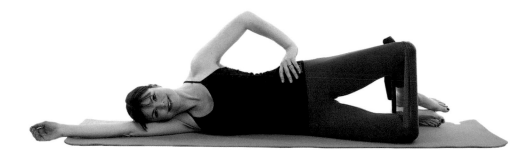

Single leg bridge

- Lie on your back with your feet and knees hip-width apart (A).

- Exhale, engage navel to spine and use your glutes to lift your hips up in the air so that you form a straight line from your knee to hip to shoulder (B).

- Inhale and keep a neutral spine and your pelvis level.

- Exhale to lift one foot off the floor (C). Inhale to place it back down maintaining a level pelvis throughout.

- Work alternate sides for 10 reps each.

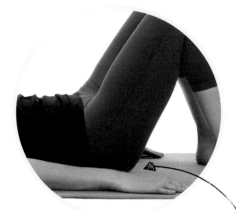

Keep your tail bone slightly tucked under to prevent your lower back from arching.

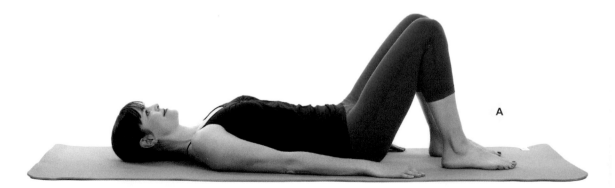

A

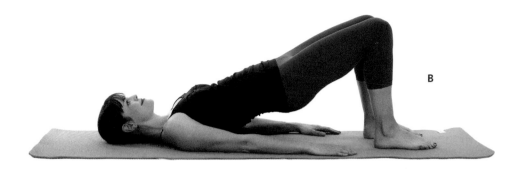

B

TO PROGRESS

- Lift your hips up as before, then lift your right leg to a table top (C).

- Lower and lift your hips up and down eight to 10 times working the left glute/hamstring.

- Replace your foot to the floor and lower your hips back down.

- Repeat on the other side for eight to 10 times.

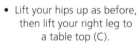

Imagine you have a spirit level on your hips to help you stay level.

If you feel that your hamstring might cramp, stop and stretch.

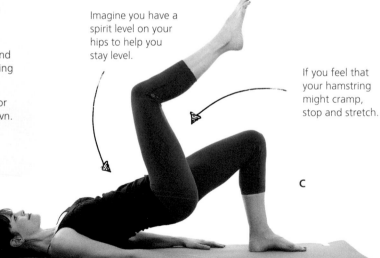

C

Heel squeeze prone

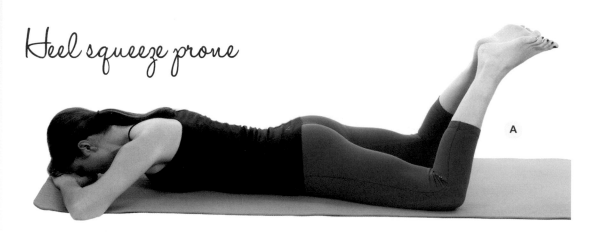

- Lie face down with your forehead supported on the back of your hands.

- Take your legs wide apart and bend your knees, bringing your heels together like a frog's legs (A).

- Keep your spine in neutral by slightly tucking your tail bone under by pressing your pubic bone into the mat and keep your core engaged.

- Inhale to prepare.

- Exhale and squeeze your heels together, squeezing your bottom tightly (B).

- Repeat eight long, slow breaths.

- To increase the intensity, lengthen your knees off the floor as you squeeze (C).

Keep your spine in neutral throughout and your abdominals drawn in.

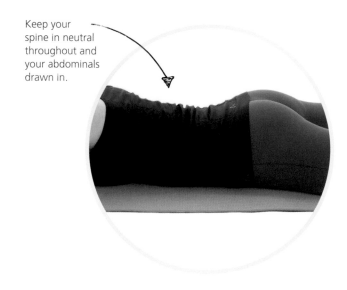

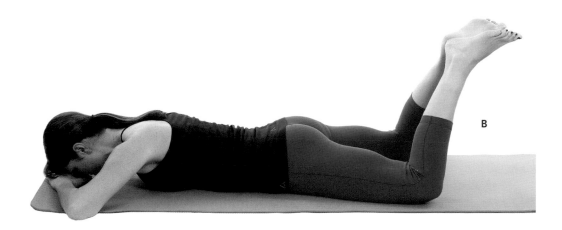

B

Think of lengthening through the front of your thighs as you squeeze.

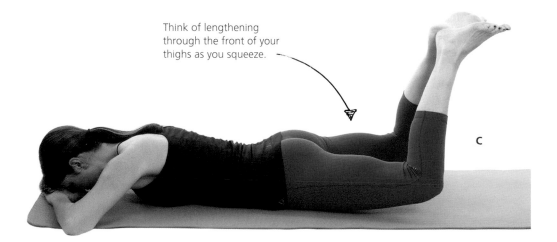

C

10-minute bum workout

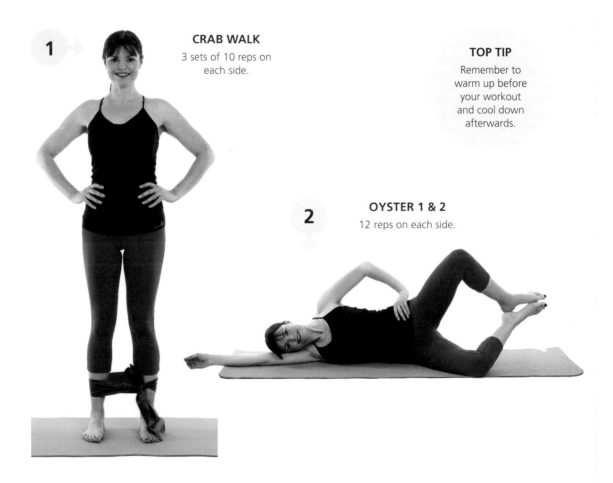

1 →

CRAB WALK

3 sets of 10 reps on each side.

TOP TIP

Remember to warm up before your workout and cool down afterwards.

2

OYSTER 1 & 2

12 reps on each side.

3 **SINGLE LEG BRIDGE**
10 reps on each side.

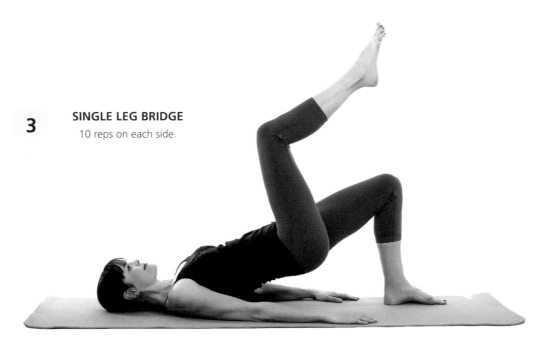

4 **HEEL SQUEEZE PRONE**
8 breaths.

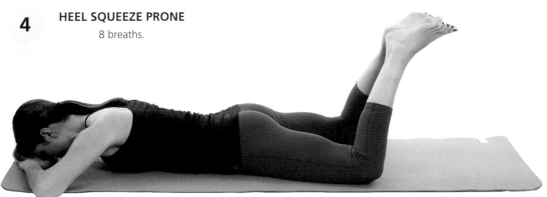

CHAPTER 3

Amazing Arms

Modern life is enough to give you a hunched back. Sitting at computers, hunching over portable devices or being in the car for hours on end is ageing us prematurely and giving us rounded shoulders and curved backs – not to mention headaches, stiff necks and sore shoulders!

This chapter focuses on counteracting these negative postures.

You will open your shoulders and chest and lengthen and strengthen your upper back and shoulder muscles. We'll also target the global 'mover' muscles of the shoulders and arms to help create tone and definition.

Goodbye bingo wings!

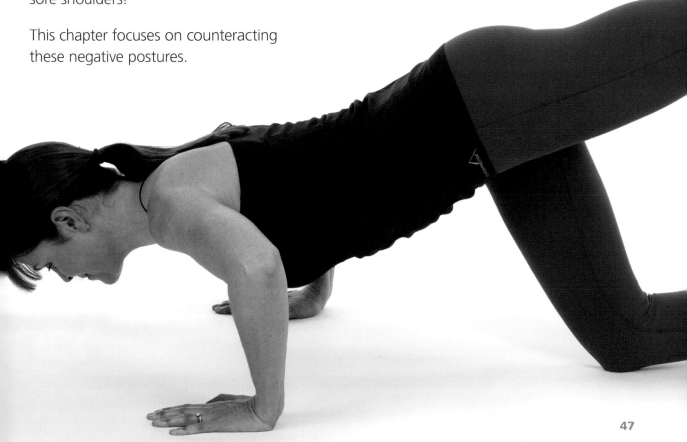

Dumb waiter

- Stand with feet hip-width apart, elbows touching your waist and bent to a right angle with your palms facing up.

- Exhale and gently draw your navel in towards your spine (A).

- Inhale as you slowly move your hands apart while working the muscles between your shoulder blades.

- Keep your forearms parallel to the floor throughout (B).

- Exhale to move your hands back to the start position.

- Repeat eight times.

Keep your spine and pelvis in neutral.

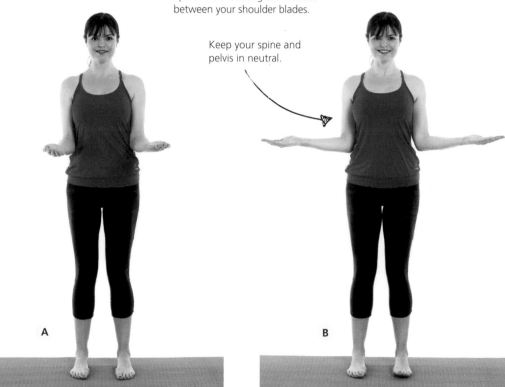

A

B

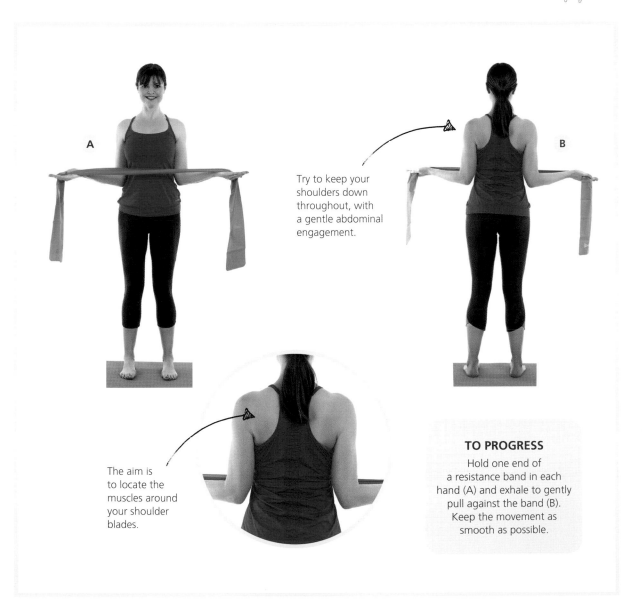

A

Try to keep your shoulders down throughout, with a gentle abdominal engagement.

B

The aim is to locate the muscles around your shoulder blades.

TO PROGRESS

Hold one end of a resistance band in each hand (A) and exhale to gently pull against the band (B). Keep the movement as smooth as possible.

Cat twist

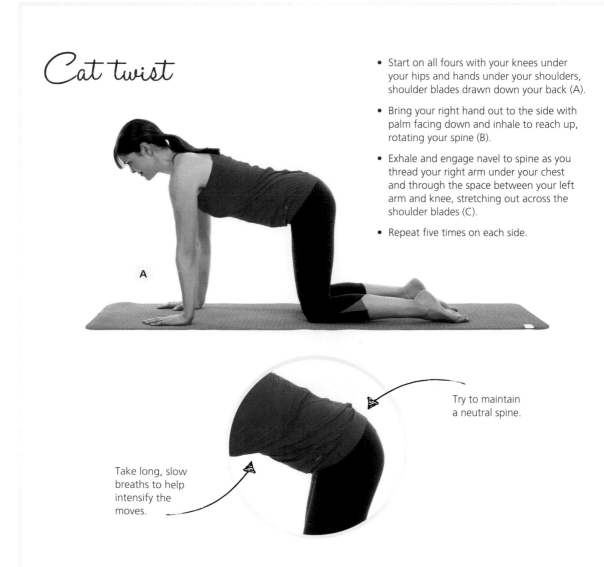

- Start on all fours with your knees under your hips and hands under your shoulders, shoulder blades drawn down your back (A).

- Bring your right hand out to the side with palm facing down and inhale to reach up, rotating your spine (B).

- Exhale and engage navel to spine as you thread your right arm under your chest and through the space between your left arm and knee, stretching out across the shoulder blades (C).

- Repeat five times on each side.

A

Try to maintain a neutral spine.

Take long, slow breaths to help intensify the moves.

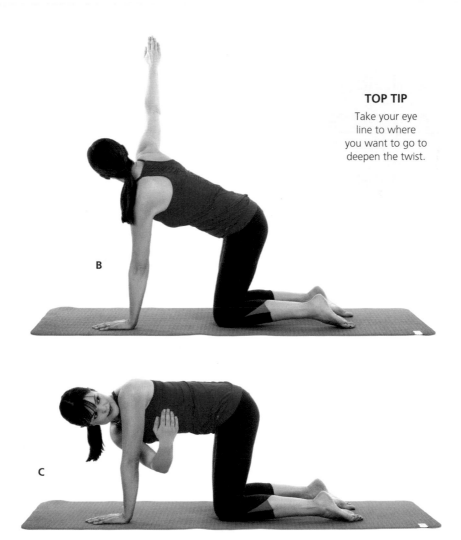

B

TOP TIP
Take your eye
line to where
you want to go to
deepen the twist.

C

Triceps with band

- Kneel up with a neutral spine and drop the resistance band behind you with your right arm.

- Take hold of the other end with your left hand, ensuring there is some tension in the band (A).

- Keeping your left hand firmly in the small of your back, inhale to prepare.

- Exhale and straighten your right arm up over your head, pulling on the band (B).

- Inhale and slowly bend your arm back down.

- Repeat 12 times on each arm.

Keep your eye-line straight ahead and your shoulders open.

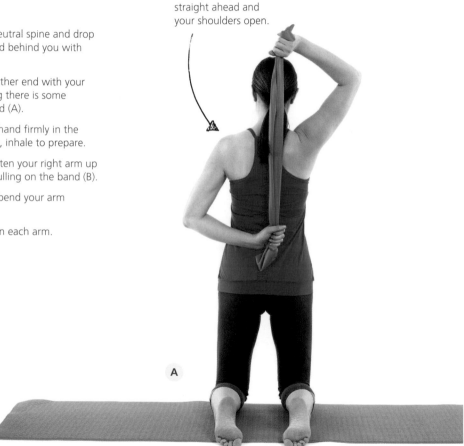

A

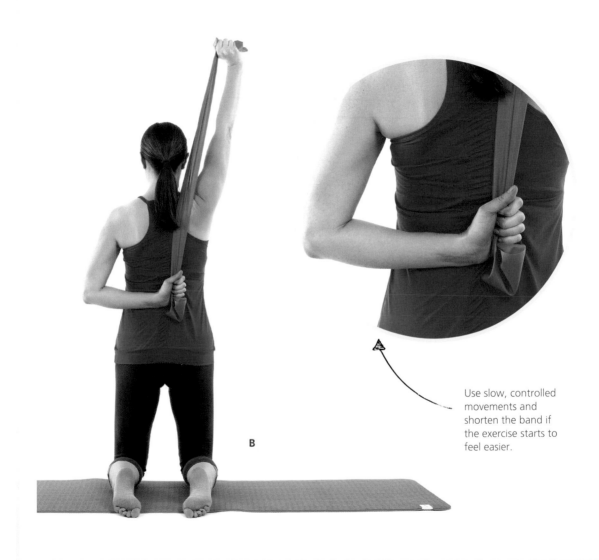

B

Use slow, controlled movements and shorten the band if the exercise starts to feel easier.

Arms ab curl

- Lie on your back with your knees bent and your feet and knees hip-width apart, with a light dumbbell or a bottle of water in each hand (A).

- Exhale, engage navel to spine and curl your head and shoulders off the mat, lifting your arms off the floor with a slightly bent elbow (B).

- Keep your head and shoulders up as you exhale to bend your elbows, bringing the weights towards your shoulders (C).

- Inhale to straighten.

- Do this 10 times.

- Bring your head and arms back to the floor and rest for a few breath cycles.

- Now exhale and lift your head and shoulders again, this time bringing your arms straight up towards the ceiling (D).

- Keeping your head and shoulders up, bend your elbows, lowering the weights down towards your ears (E).

- Do this 10 times.

- Return to the floor and gently roll your head from side to side to relax your neck.

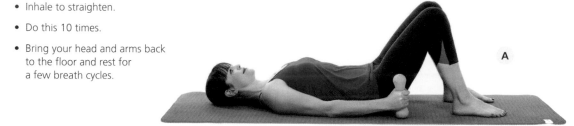

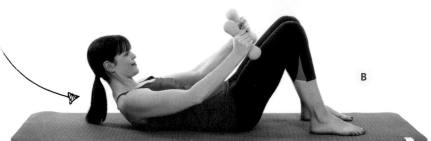

Keep your shoulders away from your ears and your shoulder blades drawn down your back.

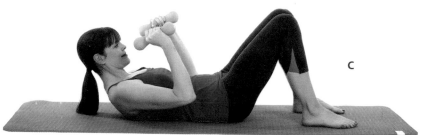

C

If you feel this is too challenging for your neck, support your head in one hand and work one arm at a time or support your head on a cushion and work both arms.

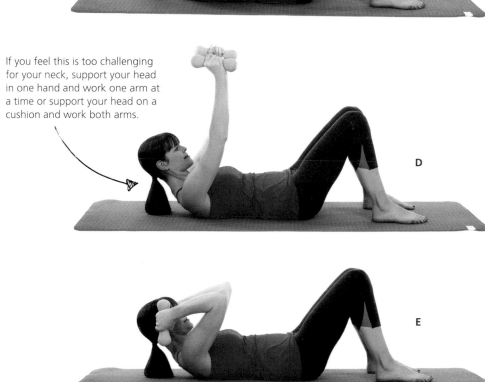

D

E

10-minute arms workout

1 → **DUMB WAITER**
8 reps.

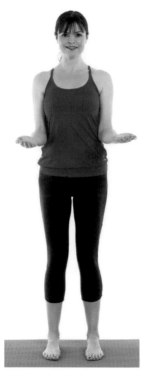

2 **CAT TWIST**
10 reps on each side.

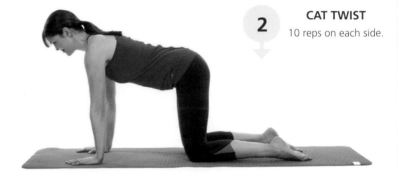

TOP TIP
Don't push your body too hard. If you are finding the exercises difficult, it's ok to stop.

TRICEPS WITH BAND
3
12 reps on each arm.

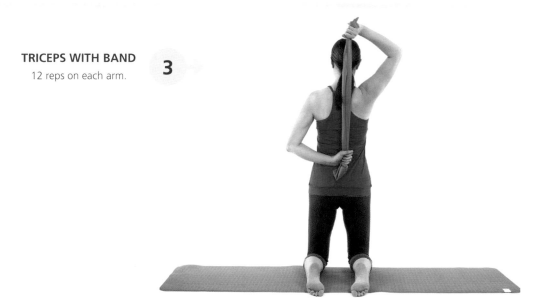

4
ARMS AB CURL
10 reps biceps and
10 reps triceps.

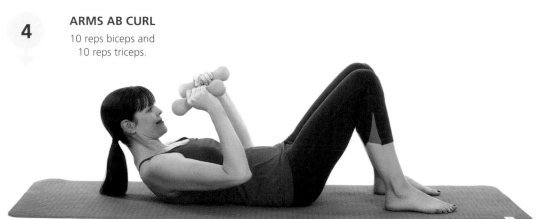

CHAPTER 4

Lean Legs

This chapter is all about creating the illusion of longer, leaner legs. You can't make your legs longer than you were blessed with, but by improving your posture and exercising the right way, you can make yourself look taller and you can slim your hips and thighs to enhance the effect.

These exercises only use the weight of your body so they tighten and tone rather than build your muscles. They work on both the large 'global' muscles of the hips and thighs and the smaller 'local' muscles, helping to tighten and pull up in your buttocks and outer hips.

You will often be asked to 'lengthen and lift' the legs instead of 'lift'. This is important. Take, for example, the side leg lift exercise. Try lying on your side and just lift and lower the leg. Now perform the exercise following the instructions and teaching tips carefully, lengthening your leg from the waist to the toe – just feel the difference it makes!

Scooter

Keep your stationary knee completely still with it over and in line with your second toe.

- Stand with your feet hip-width apart and parallel.
- Bend both knees, keeping your back straight and your abs in.
- Shift your weight on to your right leg so that your left foot/toe rests very lightly on the floor (A).
- Inhale to prepare.
- Exhale, engage your abs and lengthen your leg behind you (B).
- Inhale to return.
- Perform 15 reps on each side.

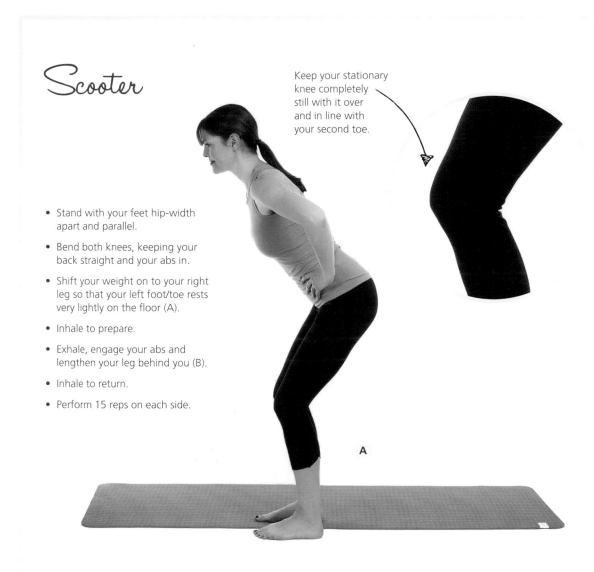

A

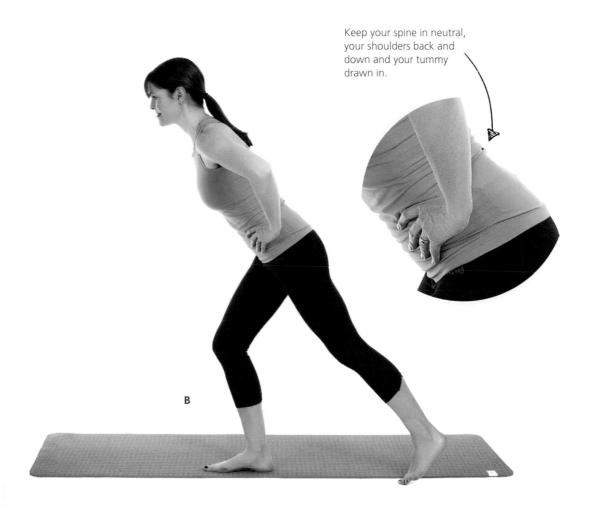

Keep your spine in neutral, your shoulders back and down and your tummy drawn in.

B

Plié squat

- Stand with your feet wide apart and your toes pointing outwards.

- Place your hands on your hips and draw your shoulders back and down (A).

- Inhale and bend your knees out wide over your toes (B).

- Exhale and squeeze your bottom as you push yourself back upright.

- Repeat this 15 times.

- Now hold in the 'down' position and lift your heels up and down 10 times (C).

- For more intensity, hold dumbbells in front of your thighs and lift them straight out to shoulder height with each plié.

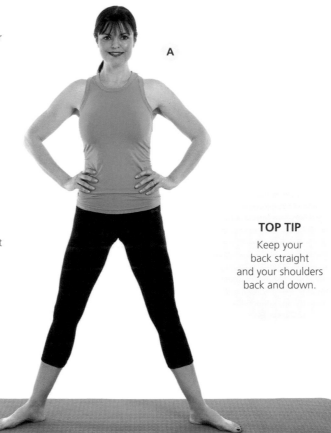

A

TOP TIP
Keep your
back straight
and your shoulders
back and down.

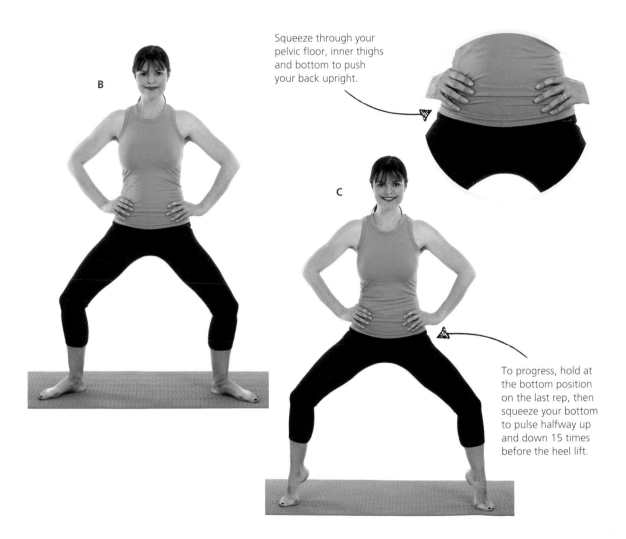

B

Squeeze through your pelvic floor, inner thighs and bottom to push your back upright.

C

To progress, hold at the bottom position on the last rep, then squeeze your bottom to pulse halfway up and down 15 times before the heel lift.

Side leg lift

- Lie on your right side with your head on your outstretched arm, your bottom leg bent and top leg out straight and raised slightly (A).

- Place your top hand on your hip and try to lengthen your waist off the floor (B).

- Exhale to lift the top leg with your foot parallel to the floor (C).

- Inhale to lower.

- Repeat the exercise 10 times with your leg turned inwards and your toes pointing towards the floor.

- Now repeat the exercise a further 10 times with your leg turned out and your toes pointing up towards the ceiling (D).

TOP TIP

For best results, slowly exhale and tighten your invisible corset each time you lift your leg.

A

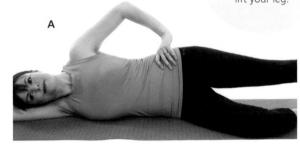

B

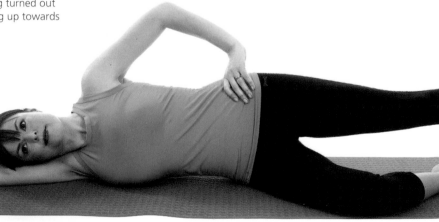

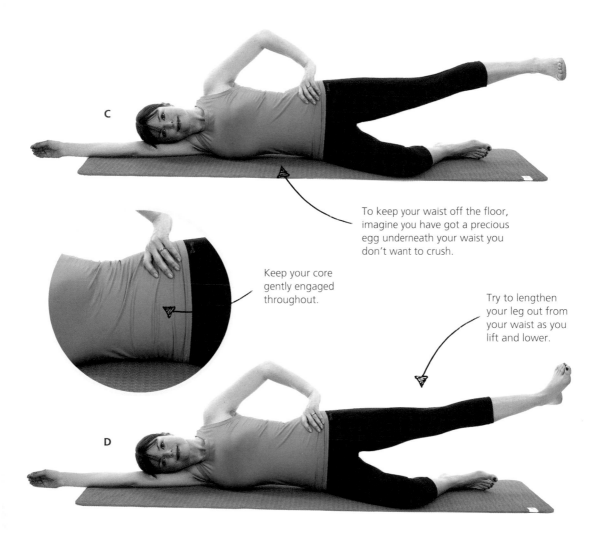

C

To keep your waist off the floor, imagine you have got a precious egg underneath your waist you don't want to crush.

Keep your core gently engaged throughout.

Try to lengthen your leg out from your waist as you lift and lower.

D

Side leg circle

- Stay on your right side as in the side leg lift on the previous page.

- This time instead of lifting your leg, stretch it out long and circle it around 10 times in each direction.

A

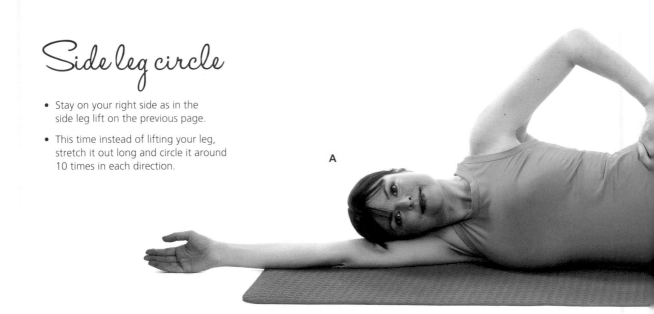

Keep your waist lengthened off the floor as with the side leg lift and reach out as though you are trying to trace the inside edge of a barrel placed just out of reach of your foot.

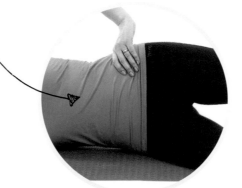

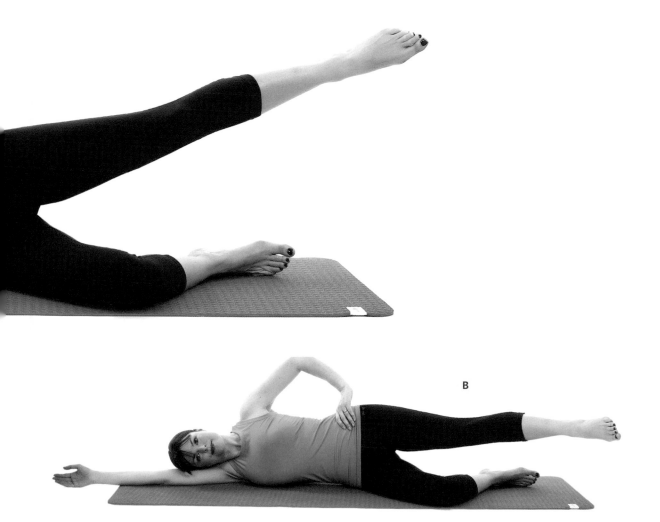

B

10-minute leg workout

1 → **SCOOTER**
15 reps on each side.

2 → **PLIÉ SQUAT**
15 reps.

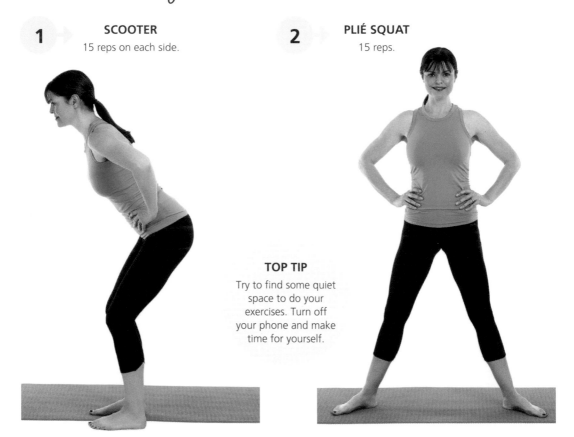

TOP TIP
Try to find some quiet space to do your exercises. Turn off your phone and make time for yourself.

3 **SIDE LEG LIFT**
5 sets of 10 reps on
each side.

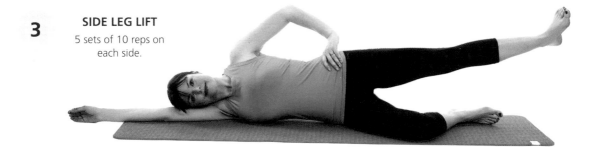

4 **SIDE LEG CIRCLE**
10 reps in each direction
on both sides.

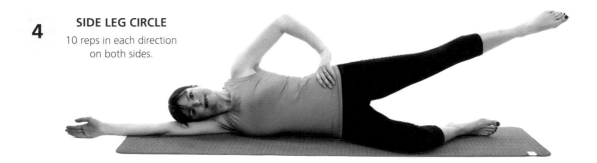

CHAPTER 5

Flat Abs

When asked which part of their body they would like to improve, many people say their abs, tummy, waist, love handles or muffin top. Our mid-sections are a problem area due to too much body fat, poor posture and weak tummy muscles. Pilates will not significantly reduce body fat – this is where a balanced routine with some cardiovascular exercise and a

healthy diet are needed – but it will give you great abdominal tone, better posture and a flatter mid-section.

All Pilates exercises start by engaging your centre, so this book will help you work towards a stronger core and better abs. The more you practise Pilates, the more natural the moves will become when you use its principles in your everyday life, enhancing the effect on your core.

Roll up (band beginners)

- Sit up tall with your legs bent and a resistance band wrapped around your feet while holding the ends in your hands (A).

- Exhale and draw navel to spine as you tilt your pelvis and begin rolling half way back towards the floor (B).

- Inhale and roll back up keeping your abs drawn in.

- Repeat five to eight times.

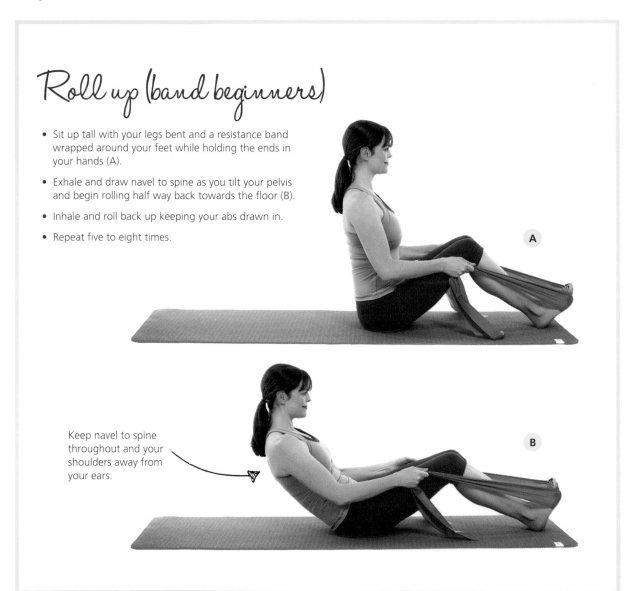

Keep navel to spine throughout and your shoulders away from your ears.

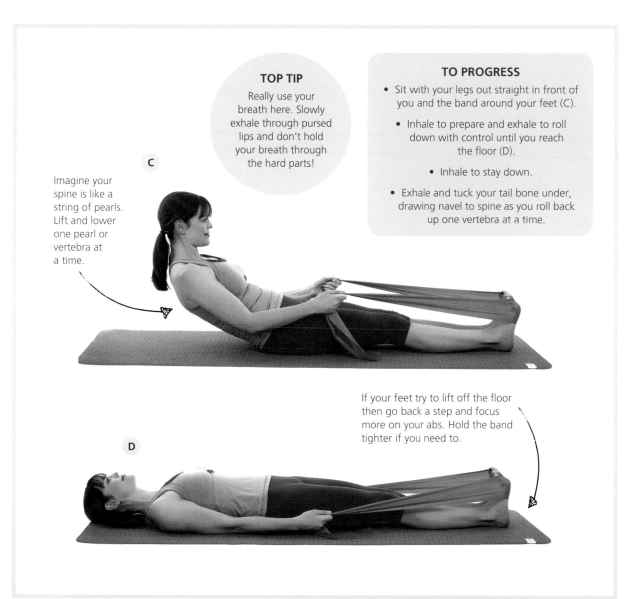

TOP TIP

Really use your breath here. Slowly exhale through pursed lips and don't hold your breath through the hard parts!

TO PROGRESS

- Sit with your legs out straight in front of you and the band around your feet (C).

- Inhale to prepare and exhale to roll down with control until you reach the floor (D).

- Inhale to stay down.

- Exhale and tuck your tail bone under, drawing navel to spine as you roll back up one vertebra at a time.

C

Imagine your spine is like a string of pearls. Lift and lower one pearl or vertebra at a time.

D

If your feet try to lift off the floor then go back a step and focus more on your abs. Hold the band tighter if you need to.

Scissor legs

- Lie on your back with your knees bent and your feet and knees hip-width apart.

- Exhale to bring one leg at a time up to a table-top position (A).

- Exhale to lift your head and shoulders and straighten both legs up towards the ceiling as much as you can (B).

- Inhale to prepare. Exhale and lower your left leg towards the floor for two beats then quickly switch legs (C).

- Then scissor in a fast but controlled motion, exhaling for two beats each time for 16 reps – eight on each side.

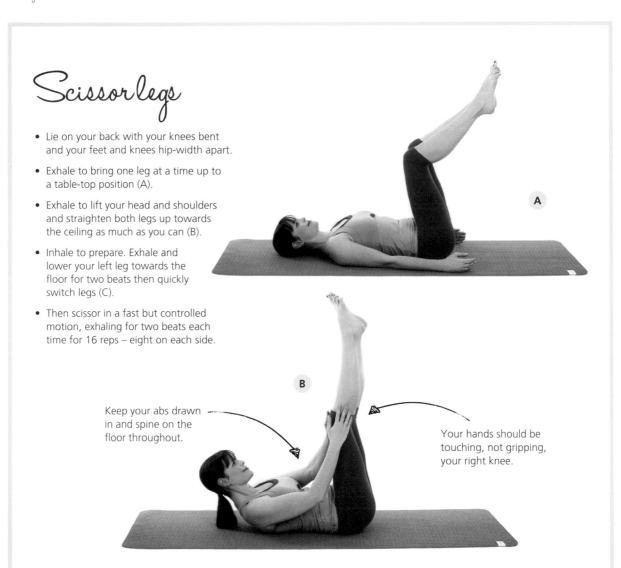

Keep your abs drawn in and spine on the floor throughout.

Your hands should be touching, not gripping, your right knee.

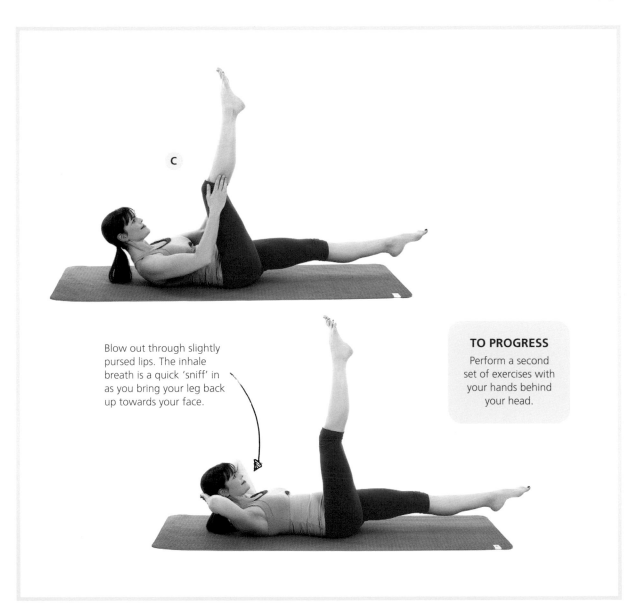

C

Blow out through slightly pursed lips. The inhale breath is a quick 'sniff' in as you bring your leg back up towards your face.

TO PROGRESS
Perform a second set of exercises with your hands behind your head.

Criss-cross

- Lie on your back with your knees bent and feet hip-width apart.

- Exhale to bring each leg one at a time up to the table-top position.

- Take your hands behind your head and exhale, engaging navel to spine to lift your head and shoulders off the floor (A).

- Inhale to prepare.

- Exhale and peel your left shoulder across towards your right hip as you extend your left leg out. Keep it as low as you can while keeping your stomach flat and your back flat and still (B).

- Inhale and move back to the centre then exhale in the opposite direction.

- Repeat 12 slow repetitions followed by 16 fast, but controlled, reps.

Try to keep your stomach flat throughout and move in a controlled manner. Don't let your hips rock as you move.

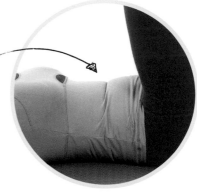

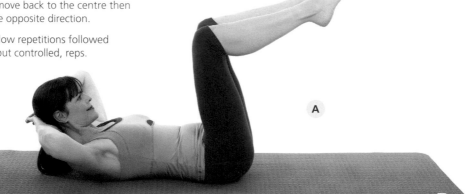

A

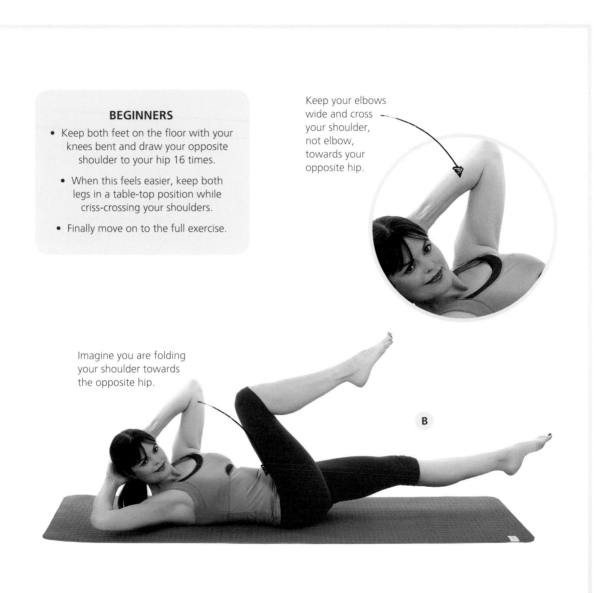

BEGINNERS

- Keep both feet on the floor with your knees bent and draw your opposite shoulder to your hip 16 times.

- When this feels easier, keep both legs in a table-top position while criss-crossing your shoulders.

- Finally move on to the full exercise.

Keep your elbows wide and cross your shoulder, not elbow, towards your opposite hip.

Imagine you are folding your shoulder towards the opposite hip.

B

Plank

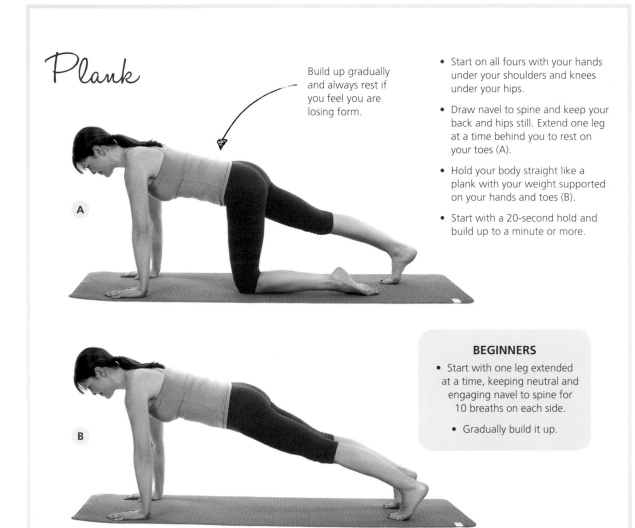

Build up gradually and always rest if you feel you are losing form.

- Start on all fours with your hands under your shoulders and knees under your hips.

- Draw navel to spine and keep your back and hips still. Extend one leg at a time behind you to rest on your toes (A).

- Hold your body straight like a plank with your weight supported on your hands and toes (B).

- Start with a 20-second hold and build up to a minute or more.

A

B

BEGINNERS

- Start with one leg extended at a time, keeping neutral and engaging navel to spine for 10 breaths on each side.

- Gradually build it up.

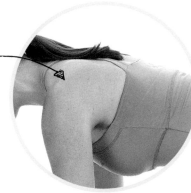

Keep your shoulders away from your ears and your head in line with your spine.

TO PROGRESS

Lift one foot at a time from the floor, maintaining a stable and level pelvis (C).

C

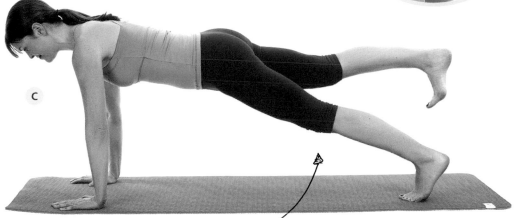

Slightly tuck your tail bone under and squeeze your glutes, draw your abs in and lock your knees, pulling your kneecaps up your thighs.

10-minute abs workout

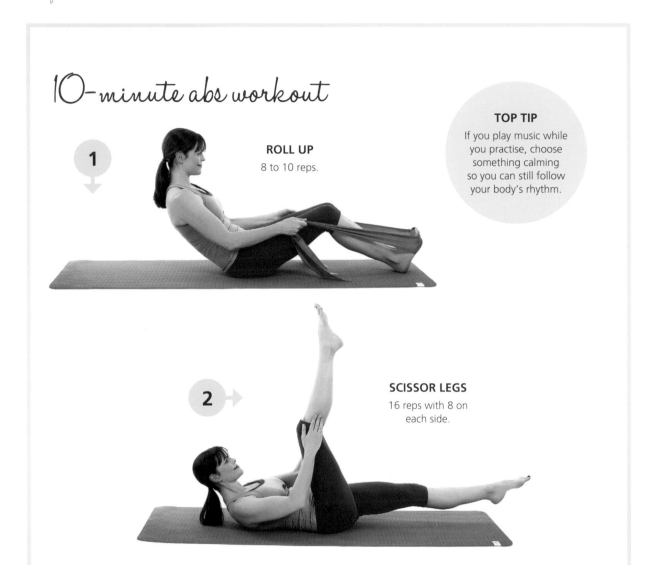

1

ROLL UP
8 to 10 reps.

TOP TIP
If you play music while you practise, choose something calming so you can still follow your body's rhythm.

2

SCISSOR LEGS
16 reps with 8 on each side.

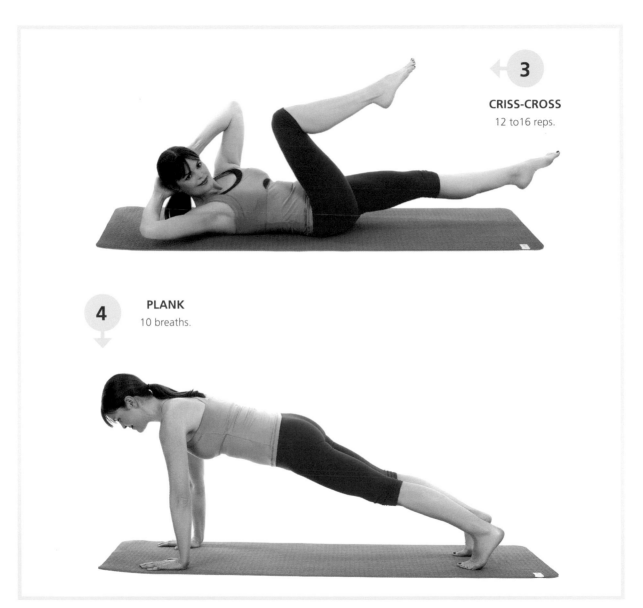

3

CRISS-CROSS
12 to16 reps.

4

PLANK
10 breaths.

CHAPTER 6

Strong Back

A healthy back is supple and strong and Pilates improves both. Your spine is designed to move through flexion (bending forwards), extension (moving backwards) and rotation (moving sideways and twisting), but we tend to sit or stand with our spines in flexion (sofa slump!). As the spine moves, it draws fluid in and out of the vertebral discs, helping to keep them plump and healthy. Lack of movement does the opposite and can age your spine, making you stiff and prone to pain. When you practise Pilates, lengthen your spine, drawing your head away from your tail bone, decompressing your spine and aiding the movement of fluid.

These exercises work both the global muscles and local stabilising ones. If you have a back condition, practise the basic exercises for a few weeks to help build stability.

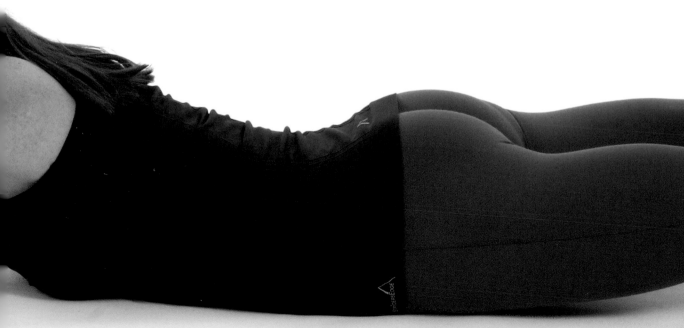

Cat stretch

- Begin on all fours in neutral spine with your hands under your shoulders, elbow creases facing each other and your knees under your hips (A).

- Inhale to prepare. Exhale, draw navel to spine and tuck your tail bone under, articulating through your spine one vertebra at a time from your tail to your head (B).

- Take a breath deep and wide into the sides of your ribs and hold the position.

- Exhale and articulate the spine from the tail bone to the head finishing with the head and upper spine slightly lifted (C).

- Repeat the exercise three times.

- Reverse the direction of articulation, head then tail bone, for three more reps.

A

Imagine a balloon inflating between each vertebra as you move, creating space and lengthening your spine.

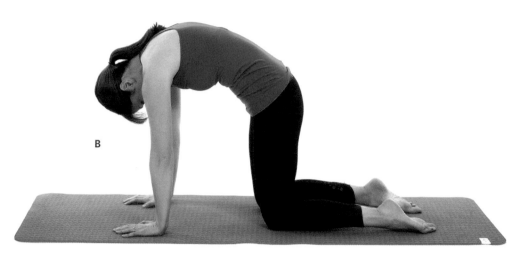

B

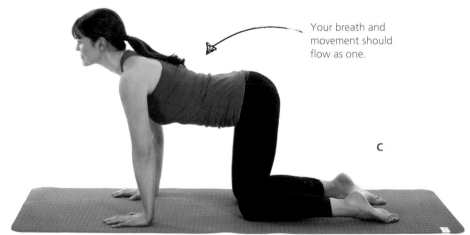

Your breath and movement should flow as one.

C

Balance hold

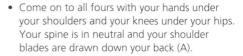

- Come on to all fours with your hands under your shoulders and your knees under your hips. Your spine is in neutral and your shoulder blades are drawn down your back (A).

- Inhale to prepare.

- Exhale, engage navel to spine and slide your right leg and left arm away from your centre until they hover off the floor. Keep your hips and back still and level (B).

- Inhale and return to the centre. Exhale and extend your other arm and leg.

- Do this 12 times. In the final rep, hold your extended position for five breaths, keeping your core tight.

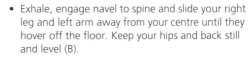

A

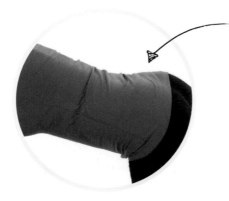

Imagine you have four glasses of water sitting on the four corners of your spine – make sure you don't spill a drop!

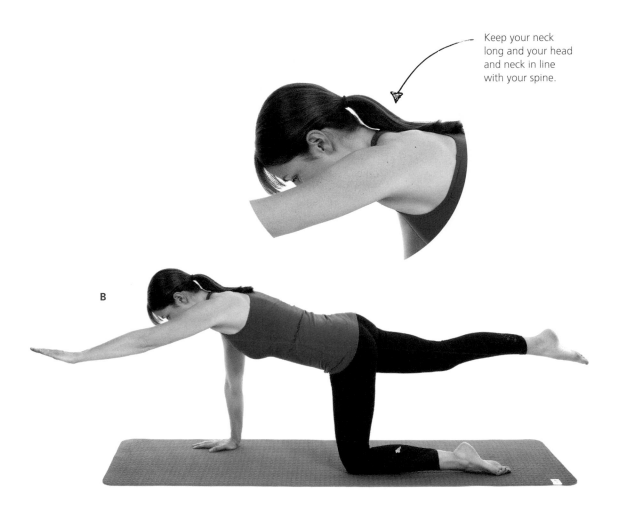

Keep your neck long and your head and neck in line with your spine.

B

Bridge

- Lie on your back in neutral spine with your knees bent and feet and knees hip-width apart.

- Inhale to prepare.

- Exhale and draw navel to spine, tucking your tail bone to tilt your pelvis (A).

- Inhale back to neutral. Exhale and tilt as above, this time articulating a couple of your vertebra off the floor (B).

- Inhale back.

- Exhale and roll one vertebra at a time off the floor until you make a straight line from your knee-to-hip-to-shoulder (C).

- Inhale to stay up and exhale to come back down one vertebra at a time.

- Repeat the exercise three to five times.

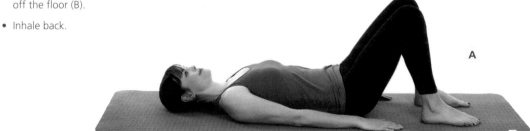

A

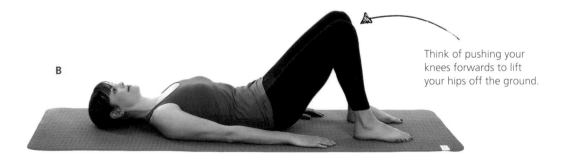

Think of pushing your knees forwards to lift your hips off the ground.

B

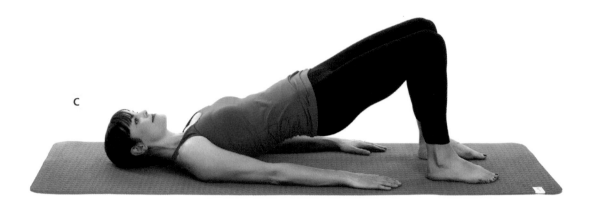

C

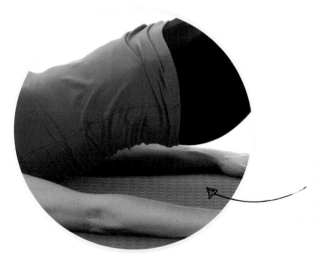

Make sure you keep your tail bone tucked under as you are lifting and at the top. You should feel the effort in your glutes and hamstrings and not your back.

Toe taps then knees to chest

- Lie on your back in neutral with knees bent and hip-width apart.

- Exhale to lift one leg at a time into the table-top position (A).

- Place your hands on your tummy with your thumbs on your bottom rib and your little fingers on your hips bones (inset).

- Inhale to prepare.

- Exhale and draw navel to spine, bringing your hips and ribs, thumb and little finger closer together as you lower one foot to tap the floor (B).

- Inhale your leg back up and continue in time with your breath for six to eight reps on each side.

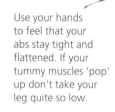

Use your hands to feel that your abs stay tight and flattened. If your tummy muscles 'pop' up don't take your leg quite so low.

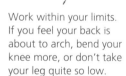

Work within your limits. If you feel your back is about to arch, bend your knee more, or don't take your leg quite so low.

A

TO PROGRESS

- As with the main exercise, but straighten your leg as you lower it (C).

ALTERNATIVE

- Place your fingertips behind your ears and flex your head and shoulders forwards.

- Exhale to lower one foot towards the floor, inhale and return as in the main exercise.

- Keep your head and shoulders lifted for 12 to 16 reps.

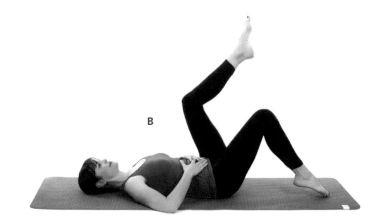

B

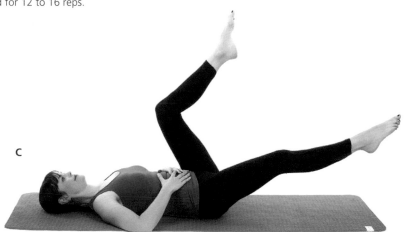

C

10-minute back workout

1

CAT
3 reps each way.

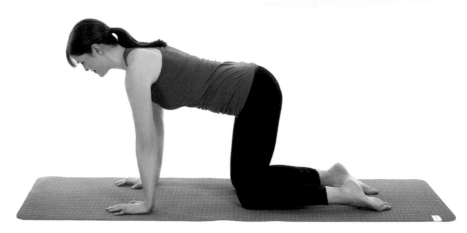

BALANCE HOLD
12 reps each side plus hold 5 breaths.

2

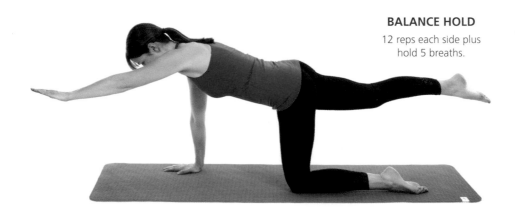

3 **BRIDGE**
5 to 8 reps.

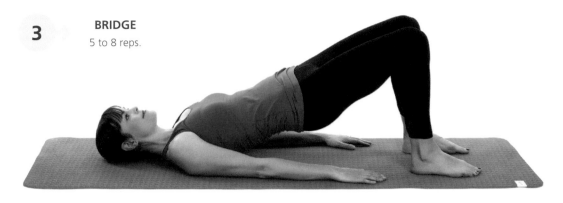

4

TOE TAPS
6 to 8 reps on
each side.

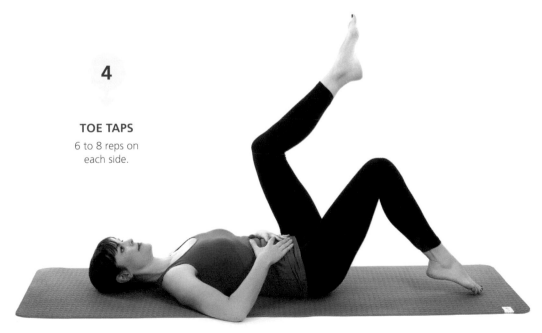

Cool Down

1   HAMSTRINGS

- Lie on your back and wrap a resistance band around your right foot.

- Straighten your right leg up towards the ceiling until you feel a stretch down the back of your thigh, gently pulling on the band to increase the stretch (A).

- Hold for several deep breaths and then swap sides.

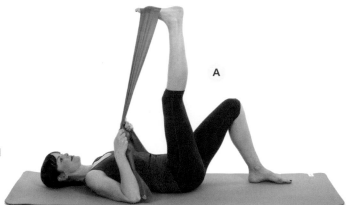

2   GLUTE STRETCH

- Stay on your back and cross your left ankle over your bent right knee.

- Draw both knees in towards your chest, then link your hands together around the back of your right thigh (A).

- Hold and take several deep breaths then change legs.

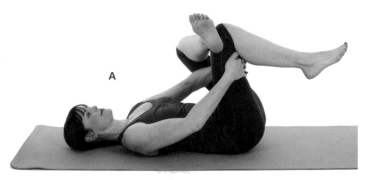

3   **SIDE TWIST**

- Lie on your back with your arms extended out at shoulder height and your knees bent.

- Slowly lower your legs over to the left, allowing your right foot to lift off the floor, and turn your head to the right (A).

- Hold for several breaths on each side and repeat the exercise two to three times.

A

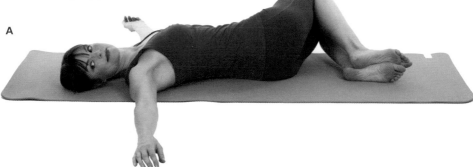

4   **HIP FLEXOR RELEASE**

- Lying on your back, draw your right knee into your chest and hold on to it with your hands.

- Lengthen your left leg out on the floor (A).

- Take three deep breaths, squeezing your right knee to your chest as you exhale and completely relaxing your left leg. This is a passive stretch for this leg.

- Repeat the exercise on the other side.

A

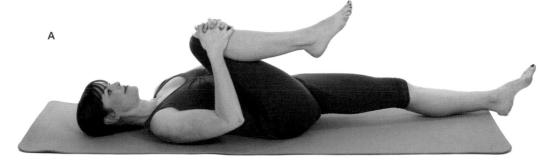

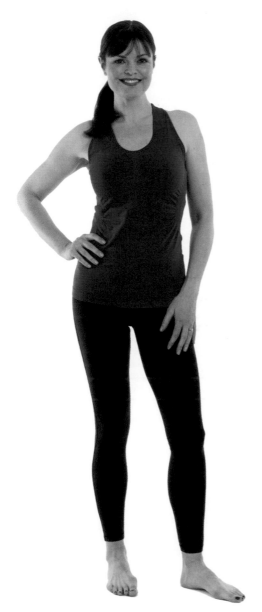

Well done

Once you have started exercising with the Pilates system, it shouldn't be long before you start to feel its benefits. Remember, 10 minutes is better than no minutes, so keep this book handy to make the most of any unexpected windows of opportunity. It is recommended that you try to do at least one 10-minute Pilates workout, five days a week.

You could do the Flat Abs workout on after a run, or do the Amazing Arms workout to energise you at lunch time. However you choose to use this book, you will continue to discover the amazing benefits of Pilates for a happier, healthier and more balanced body for life.

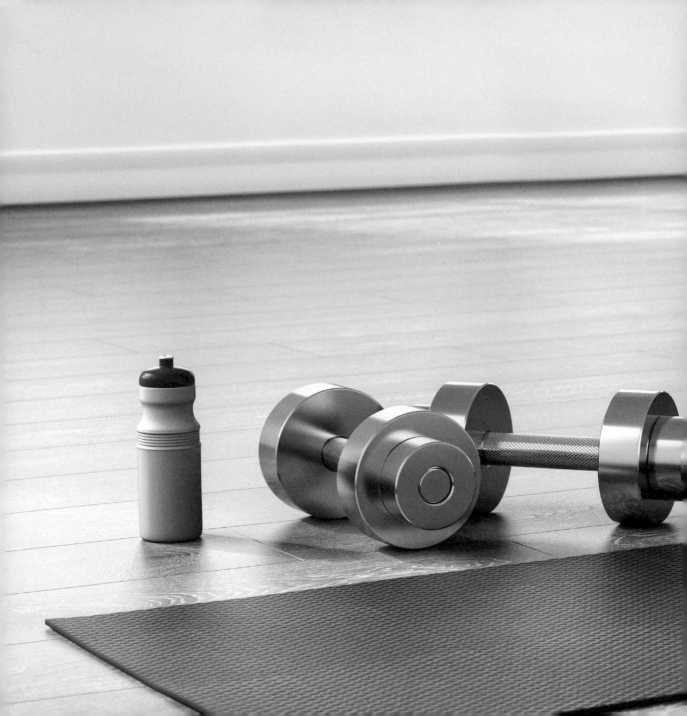